Somatic Lessons

Narrating Patienthood and Illness in Indian Medical Literature

Anthony Cerulli

SUNY PRESS

Cover photo taken from *Caraka Samhita*. Edited by Khemaraja Krishnadasa with a Hindi commentary by Mihiracandra. Mumbai: Shrivenkateshvar Press, 1898.

Published by State University of New York Press, Albany

For information, contact State University of New York Press, Albany, NY
www.sunypress.edu

Production by Kelli Williams-LeRoux
Marketing by Kate McDonnell

Library of Congress Cataloging-in-Publication Data

Cerulli, Anthony Michael.
Somatic lessons : narrating patienthood and illness in Indian medical literature / Anthony Cerulli.
pages cm. — (SUNY series in Hindu studies)
Based on the author's thesis (Ph. D.), University of Chicago, Faculty of the Divinity School, 2007.
Includes bibliographical references and index.
ISBN 978-1-4384-4387-4 (hardcover : alk. paper)
1. Medicine, Ayurvedic—History. 2. Medical literature—India—History and criticism. 3. Sanskrit literature—History and criticism. I. Title.

R605.C48 2012
615.5'38—dc23 2011047448

10 9 8 7 6 5 4 3 2 1

Somatic Lessons

SUNY series in Hindu Studies

Wendy Doniger, editor

For Jaview LaTulli

ഈ മനുഷ്യന്റെ ശരിയായ സുഹൃത്ത്

Contents

List of Figures

Acknowledgments

This book has been in the works for a long time. All the while, I have acquired many debts, and I am happy to begin to repay them here by thanking those people and institutions that helped me in the process of researching, writing, and editing this book. To begin, I want to thank two very important people without whom this book would never have seen the light of day. First, I am tremendously grateful to my teacher, mentor, and friend, Wendy Doniger. With dogged commitment and enthusiasm, she has directed, cheered on, corrected, inspired, and assisted my work on this project in its numerous incarnations. Wendy's unfaltering and incomparable guidance, towering yet reasonable intellectual expectations, and friendship over the years have made my studies of Sanskrit literature, South Asian religions, and storytelling both possible and exhilarating. Next, I owe an enormous debt of gratitude to Dominik Wujastyk. Always a source of sound counsel and incisive analysis, Dominik's excellent work on the history of medicine in India and Sanskrit medical literature is the touchstone for my own work in the field of Indian medical history. It is difficult to imagine how I can ever repay the generosity of intellect, time, and spirit I owe to these two people.

For their advice, generosity, and patience over the years, I am grateful to the following people as well. Tracy Pintchman, my *ādiguru*, moved me with her vast knowledge of South Asian religions while I was a young, somewhat adrift college student. She was then and continues to be an important role model for me as a teacher and scholar. Matthew Kapstein's keen insight and direction in the early stages of my work on the history of medicine and religions in India helped me to articulate and sustain the central argument of this book. I am enormously grateful to Kunal and Shubhra Chakrabarti, who have always opened their home to me whenever I am in Delhi. Kunal's advice about the mythology of Jātahāriṇī, discussed in Chapter 4, while I was a grad student at the University of Chicago, was instrumental in the development of this project. I would also like to thank Dr. S. K. Shukla, at Jawaharlal Nehru University, who sat with me for hours every day during the searing Delhi summer of 2005, wading through some of the knottier parts of Ānandarāya's *nāṭaka*, which I discuss in Chapter 6.

Several people helped me in the process of doing the research that went into this book. In Thiruvananthapuram, I would like to thank P. J. Cherian of the Kerala Council for Historical Research and my Malayalam teacher, Dr. V. K. Bindu of Kerala University. Additionally, I extend a most emphatic thank you to everyone at Valloor Mana and Ullanoor Mana: Shankaran Namboothiri, Brahmadathan Namboothiri, Vimala Antarjanam, Dr. Madhu K. P., Dr. Vijith Sasidhar, Dr. Sreejith K. J., and Parvathy U. M. T. The importance of their hospitality, instruction, and friendship over the years is beyond measure. Moreover, I owe a great deal of thanks to Tsutomu Yamashita, my colleague and friend from Kyoto who introduced me to everyone at Valloor Mana and Ullanoor Mana and who inspired me with his interest in the history and practice of medicine in Kerala.

Special thanks are also owed to a few of the people who helped me gather materials for this book. In particular, I am grateful to P. L. Shaji of the Oriental Research Institute and Manuscript Library at Kerala University; without his generosity of time and energy in obtaining Malayalam and Sanskrit manuscripts this project would never have taken off. P. Ram Manohar of the AVT Institute for Advanced Research in Coimbatore not only was integral in helping me to gather materials, especially an important, early edition of the *Jīvānandanam*, but he also instilled in me an appreciation for learning to read and understand the medical literature on its own terms, as the compilers of the texts suggest the literature should be read and understood. I thank Philipp Maas for leading me to the terrific artwork that is on the cover of this book. And finally, I would like to thank Dan Mulvey of the Warren Hunting Smith Library at Hobart and William Smith Colleges, who tracked down countless resources for me over the past two years.

I am thankful to the many people who helped me revise and prepare this book for publication. Kenneth G. Zysk read the entire manuscript and made countless useful comments and suggestions. Sarah Berry introduced me to important theories and methods in the medical humanities that have greatly improved this work and made possible future projects. I am also grateful to the three anonymous reviewers for their many useful suggestions, corrections, and encouraging nudges to shape the book into its present form. And I am extremely grateful to my fantastic editors at the State University of New York Press, Nancy Ellegate, Kelli Williams-LeRoux, Emily Keneston, and Eileen Nizer.

Several institutions and foundations supported my research and writing, and to them I am very thankful. An American Council of Learned Societies ACLS/SSRC/NEH International and Area Studies Fellowship in 2011–12 was instrumental in bringing this book to publication. I also received support from the U.S. Department of Education Fulbright-Hays DDRA program, the Martin Marty Center of the University of Chicago Divinity School, the Committee on Southern Asian Studies at the University of Chicago, and a Faculty Research Grant from Hobart and William Smith Colleges. At the Colleges, I would also like to thank former Provost, Teresa Amott, and the three alternating chairs of my department, Michael Dobkowski, Susan Henking, and Richard Salter, each of whom has enthusiastically supported my work. I owe an extra-special thank you to everyone at the Wellcome Trust Centre for the History of Medicine at the University College London, who generously hosted me on two extended periods of research. And thank you to Routledge for permission to reprint portions of Chapter 4, which appeared as "Calculating Fecundity in the *Kāśyapa Saṃhitā*" in Fabrizio Ferrari's *Health and Religious Rituals in South Asia* (2011).

Many thanks are owed to my friends outside academia for their encouragement and camaraderie throughout the various stages of this project. In particular, I extend hearty thanks to Peter Heath, Andy Korczynski, Scott Mersy, and Bill Warshaw. Whether they realize it or not, each of them has, in his own inimitable, typically unspoken, but sometimes candid way, helped me move this project along.

A special word of appreciation also goes to my parents, Jill and Louis Cerulli, who have been an endless source of support, encouragement, and sage advice for many years. They have been patient and understanding beyond all expectations throughout it all, and I cannot thank them enough. My brother, Buck, also has been helpful during this project, occasionally reading drafts of my writing and always pointing me in profitable directions for further study. Thanks also to my mother-in-law, Mary Ann Javier, for her constant interest in what I have been doing and for regularly expressing her delight as I progress along my academic career.

Finally, this book could not have begun, developed, or reached completion without the enduring support and patience of my wife, Gabrielle Javier-Cerulli. She has been many important things to me as I researched and wrote this book: editor, critic, cheerleader, therapist, among other things. For her help and willingness to put up with me and this project, I am forever grateful. To my son, Arlo Loubuck Cerulli, thank you for lightening my spirits during the past five years and for restoring my sense of humor at all the right times. And last, to the truly greatest dog a guy could ever have, Macey, there is no way I can repay you for the incomparable and unconditional companionship you have given me.

Abbreviations

AB	*Aitareya Brāhmaṇa*
AHS	*Aṣṭāṅgahṛdayasaṃhitā*
AP	*Agni Purāṇa*
AŚ	*Arthaśāstra*
ASS	*Aṣṭāṅgasaṃgrahasaṃhitā*
AV	*Atharvaveda*
BG	*Bhagavadgītā*
BhP	*Bhāgavata Purāṇa*
BrāP	*Brahmā Purāṇa*
BṛhS	*Bṛhatsaṃhitā*
BrṇḍP	*Brahmāṇḍa Purāṇa*
BS	*Bhelasaṃhitā*
BVP	*Bhāvaprakāśa*
Ci	Cikitsāsthāna
CS	*Carakasaṃhitā*
GP	*Garuḍa Purāṇa*
HIML	*A History of Indian Medical Literature*
Ind	Indriyasthāna
JVM	*Jīvānandanam*
KauS	*Kauśika Sūtra*
KālP	*Kālikā Purāṇa*
Kp	Kalpasthāna
KP	*Kūrma Purāṇa*
KS	*Kāśyapasaṃhitā*
KṭhS	*Kāṭhakasaṃhitā*
Manu	*Manusmṛti*
MāP	*Mārkaṇḍeya Purāṇa*
MBh	*Mahābhārata*
MN	*Mādhavanidāna*
MP	*Matsya Purāṇa*

MS	*Maitrāyaṇīsaṃhitā*
Ni	Nidānasthāna
PP	*Padma Purāṇa*
RĀM	*Rāmāyaṇa*
ṚV	*Ṛgveda*
Śā	Śārīrasthāna
ŚB	*Śatapatha Brāhmaṇa*
Si	Siddhisthāna
ŚP	*Śiva Purāṇa*
SS	*Suśrutasaṃhitā*
Sū	Sūtrasthāna
TS	*Taittirīyasaṃhitā*
Ut	Uttaratantra or Uttarasthāna
VāP	*Vāyu Purāṇa*
Vi	Vimānasthāna
VP	*Viṣṇu Purāṇa*
YS	*Yājñavalkyasmṛti*
YV	*Yajurveda*

Note on Transliteration, Pronunciation, and Translation

All transliterations from Sanskrit and Hindi in the body of the text are in italics and follow standard lexicographical usage. By and large, Sanskrit pronunciation is very similar to pronunciation in Italian: vowels are open (i.e., they are pronounced by opening the mouth wide and holding the tongue low inside the mouth), and consonants carry the same sound wherever they occur. Below is a general guide to the pronunciation of Sanskrit vowels (including diphthongs) and a handful of perhaps unfamiliar-sounding consonants for the native English speaker that appear in the following pages:

a	pronounced like the u in "but"
ā	pronounced like the a in "father"
ai	pronounced like the y in "spry"
au	pronounced like the ou in "cloud"
c	pronounced like the ch in "cheese"
e	pronounced like the a in "skate"
g	pronounced like the g in "go"
i	pronounced like the i in "pick"
ī	pronounced like the ee in "street"
ṅ	pronounced like the n in "zing"
ñ	pronounced like the n in "venue"
o	pronounced like the o in "vote"
ph	pronounced like the p in "pin"
ṛ	pronounced like the ri in "sprig"
ś and ṣ	pronounced like the sh in "shimmy"
u	pronounced like the initial u in "future"
ū	pronounced like the oo in "drool"

A dot underneath a letter—ṭ, ṭh, ḍ, ḍh, ṇ—signals a retroflex consonant. The retroflex is a uniquely Indian sound, with no express equivalent in English. To pronounce retroflexes, the tip of the tongue is curled back to the roof of the mouth when saying these letters.

All translations in this book are my own, unless otherwise noted. All editions of primary sources used in this book are listed in the bibliography.

Chapter 1

Introduction

Narrativizing the Body

Everyone gets sick. Physical and mental fluctuations between wellness and illness are par for the course of being human. Types of illness are too numerous to count, yet the ways that people ail usually happen in three ways: psychologically, somatically, and psychosomatically. This book is about what happens in the course of becoming ill. In the following chapters I ask: In which ways are people different before and after the arrival of disease? What are the processes by which people experience the shift from health into illness? In so doing, I also untangle the thorny matter of patienthood: What are some of the characteristics that mark people as so-called patients? These are the significant, framing questions of this book. They invite particular answers insofar as this book is about illness and patienthood in India, Indian medical history, and Sanskrit literature. These areas, too, are quite expansive, so in the chapters that follow I concentrate on a specific type of literary account in Indian history and Sanskrit medical literature to explain why people get sick—namely, narrative discourse. In the literature of India's classical medical tradition, Āyurveda, the ways in which, and the reasons why, people become sick are sometimes explained through stories. The stories of Āyurveda tend to explain more than just the "hows" of bodily disorders (e.g., how does contaminated water cause diarrhea?). They also address the "whys" of illness (e.g., why me and not someone else? Why now and not the day before?). They are thus valuable lenses through which to study perceived moral and social causes of health and illness in certain cultural domains of Indian history, including of course the medical field, but also religious and political institutions. The medical narratives that I present and analzye here are for the most part mythological, with gods, goddesses, and demons as the central characters. Yet as myths are wont to do, the stories of the gods serve as models or guides for humankind. Indeed, in a Sanskrit medical narrative the activities of heavenly, nonhuman characters invariably exemplify poor decisions that create unhealthy social relations, which eventually lead to the creation of sickness and disease in the world of human beings.

Although this book is primarily about the history of Indian medical literature and religion, the ways the authors of classical ayurvedic literature explain and propose to treat illness offer fresh perspectives on notions of wellness and illness to biomedical ethics and the nascent field of narrative medical studies, both which are largely restricted to the doctor–patient exchange, questions of warrant and moral principles in medical research, and, in the case of narrative medicine, personal testimonies of illness of patients of American health care. The Sanskrit stories I discuss and analyze in this book speak to theoretical questions about the ethics of illness and what it means to be a patient in South Asia specifically, but they also have cross-cultural relevance. My analysis of the narrative portrayal of somatic change from wellness to illness in Indian medical literature reveals overlooked moral codes and religious knowledge in Indian history by probing heretofore unobserved associations between cultural institutions and actors in the formation of medical discourse. This hermeneutic approach draws on multiple disciplines in the human sciences, including medical anthropology, the history of medicine, literary criticism, and the history of religions. Procedurally, the methodology I present here, not to mention the questions about disease pathology and patienthood asked in the Sanskrit narratives themselves, may be useful to scholars working in narrative medical studies and medical ethics in regions of the world apart from South Asia. At bottom, the present study attempts to elucidate the ways in which people make use of language in the production of literature. This includes authorial awareness of past and contemporary knowledge systems and their corpora, which usually manifests in the Indian context through both subtle and overt intertextual referencing. It also includes language figuration and suggestion, in which case narrative discourse is an especially effective means to convey multiple layers of meaning. When the discursive shift from clinical to narrative discourse occurs in the Sanskrit medical sources, and stories from religious and philosophical texts are adapted to the medical framework—a shift that is apparent because of changes in literary style and subject matter—the topography of the human body ceases to be an organic montage of biophysical items and becomes a medium with which to encode symbols that reflect social mores, assumptions, and fears. As readers of this literature, we follow patients—called *rogins* in Sanskrit, literally "diseased ones"—along paths of apparent moral indiscretion. Our understanding of the ethical attitude of the medical compilers, as B. K. Matilal once wrote about the philosophical opponent in Sanskrit literature, "deepens by our understanding of not so much what it says as what it rejects."[1] In my reading, the Sanskrit medical narrative ultimately denounces the patient's choices and actions, his or her *life as lived*. This reading marks a noteworthy difference between the work I am doing on illness narratives in the Sanskrit medical idiom and the work on stories of illness in biomedicine over the past two decades by scholars like Rita Charon, Arthur Kleinman, Cheryl Mattingly, Martha Montello, and others. For these scholars, as Charon and Montello once put it, "the patients are the true ethicists."[2] In Sanskrit medical narratives, the compilers of the texts are the ethicists: they aim to generate social (in)action, while the so-called patients are literary contrivances, promoters of straw-man arguments about social, religious, and political behavior. The dramatic changes in the life of the patient in the illness narratives express an ideological conversion that any human being may experience. I argue that the compilers of the Sanskrit medical literature portray the patient in the tradition's narratives as someone who must be transformed from one among the infirm, whose behavior and intentions are flawed, to a healthy person, whose behavior and intentions exhibit social and religious integrity. Āyurveda's medical narratives have a normative thrust, in other words, that attempts to be not only therapeutically effectual but also socially and religiously determinative.

Narrative discourse is a distinctive mode of argumentation in Āyurveda. While there are many narratives in the Sanskrit medical compendia, the majority of these tend to be formulaic mythologies, typically brief honorific and invocatory paeans, rather than full-fledged stories with beginnings, middles, and ends. I am concerned with the protracted narratives, which contribute to our understanding of how and why sickness and disease affect humans and which humans are likely to become ill. The stories I discuss also provide us with insight into how the compilers of India's classical medical tradition understood health in general (*svāsthya*), the state of being free from disease (*ārogya*), and possible ways for regaining this state after becoming ill. These stories describe a kind of bioexistential arc of the patient, a life trajectory that accommodates bodily ailment and disease. Disease and bodily dysfunction in these stories are not presented as merely somatic facts to accept and treat. They are portrayed as products of poor decisions, foolhardy actions, and blatant violations of knowledge, knowledge usually pertaining to the Hindu concept of dharma (which fundamentally means "duty," although many scholars have translated the term as law, justice, religion, and righteousness).

What is special about the narrativization of a patient's body in the literature of Āyurveda? And what makes this literary process of linking a human life with disease important? For the most part, the literature of Āyurveda presupposes, rather than explicitly describes, changes from wellness to illness. In the ayurvedic sources available to us today, it is clear that the compilers of the tradition sought to present the nature of health and disease in a concise and matter-of-fact manner. The language of this literature demonstrates a kind of detached, pragmatic rationality useful to clinical reasoning. Even today in ayurvedic clinics, hospitals, and colleges in India this type of discourse serves as the basis for establishing the causes, courses, and treatments of disease and the writing of medical reports. Of course, it is a mode of discourse that is unique neither to Āyurveda nor to India, for it is also common throughout the world wherever medicine is practiced. In a pioneering publication in 1998, "In Search of the Good: Narrative Reasoning in Clinical Practice," Cheryl Mattingly labeled this kind of discourse in occupational therapy "chart talk." She described chart talk in contrast to storytelling, which she also identified as a prominent, if informal, vehicle of clinical reasoning. I contend throughout this book that the standard mode of ayurvedic discourse in the Sanskrit literature resembles what Mattingly had in mind when she coined the phrase "chart talk." For Mattingly, chart talk entails a strict impersonal rationality, or at least the presumption of a removed and objective diagnostic point of view that emphasizes pathology, symptomatology, therapy, pharmacology, and the like.[3] Most of ayurvedic discourse involves explicative and diagnostic reasoning rooted in observation, which seeks first to discover and subsequently to explain the underlying causes of disease. Akin to Mattingly's observation of chart talk in contemporary biomedical discourse, the body in Āyurveda is generally treated as a purely anatomical mechanism, isolable from the person to whom it belongs. The body in other words is separate from we might call the intangible character and qualities that constitute and contribute to the lived experiences of that body. The life the body leads, the very embodiment of the ayurvedic patient, and the ways in which a person actually becomes sick often are not described in the Sanskrit medical sources. But explanations of how people become ill—the processes that lead people from states of presumed wellness into states of patienthood—occasionally do crop up in the classical medical literature of India. When the medical authors speak of the transformation from wellness to illness as a lived experience, a discursive shift occurs in the texts when, following Mattingly, the clinical logic of chart talk gives way to the narrative logic of storytelling.

As I treat them here, both types of discourse, chart talk and narrative discourse, are found in the Sanskrit medical compendia, which themselves belong to the genre of textbook or perhaps manual. On the whole, the Sanskrit sources of Āyurveda as we have them today are, in the customary meaning of textbook, discursive volumes that conform to a standard or type widely held by theorists. But I also regard the Sanskrit sources, such as the compendia of Caraka, Suśruta, and Vāgbhaṭa, not as static descriptions or even hard-and-fast instructional manuals for botanical preparations, illness diagnosis, and therapy. Rather, they are generative, meaning-making sources of knowledge. They are meant for training physicians, of course, and accordingly they are knowledge to be taught, consumed and, importantly, re-presented again and again. The ayurvedic "textbooks" we have today, in other words, were composed to shape chart talk in the doctor–patient encounter. The medical narratives in the present study are decidedly different in structure, language, and history; they too are meant to affect the doctor–patient encounter, but in so doing, unlike chart talk, these discourses make room for the integration of other cultural domains in the medical context, such as religion, politics, ethics, and the like. Both forms of medical discourse taken up in this book—chart talk and narrative—are equally vital parts of classical Āyurveda.

A short narrative about the origin of garlic (*laśuna*) in the *Kāśyapasaṃhitā*, a medical "compendium," *saṃhitā*, attributed to the celebrated medical preceptor Kaśyapa, is illustrative of the difference between the two types of medical discourse I discuss here. In a chapter devoted entirely to the healing properties of garlic, following a perfunctory benediction to Prajāpati, Lord of Creatures, we find an origination myth for garlic, which I have summarized here:

> The god Indra gave his wife, Indrāṇī, some divine nectar to drink because she had been unable to conceive a child for one hundred years. Upon drinking the nectar, the delicate Indrāṇī promptly belched, and some of the nectar fell out of her mouth and onto the unclean ground. Thereupon Indra declared that Indrāṇī would have many sons. The nectar that fell to the earth became a rejuvenating substance (*rasāyana*) for humankind. Yet because of its inauspicious discharge in the form of a burp, and eventual setting on the ground, the nectar will have a foul smell and twice-borns shall not go near it. On earth its name will be garlic.[4]

The text then swiftly moves on to the medical uses of garlic for the treatment of ailing human bodies. The shift in discourse is evident in subject—from divine bodies to human bodies—as well as discursive style, from narrative prose to aphorism. The origin myth of garlic in the *Kāśyapasaṃhitā* occurs in two other medical treatises, the *Aṣṭāṅgahṛdayasaṃhitā* and the *Aṣṭāṅgasaṃgrahasaṃhitā*. What does this story have to do with a discussion of botanical properties for healing? The story's narration of the divine origin of garlic, its rejuvenating benefits, foul smell, and taboo for twice-born Hindus is a fine example of how narratives in the Sanskrit medical literature relate what Dominik Wujastyk has called the vertical and horizontal dimensions of human existence. The divine origin represents the vertical dimension, which, according to Wujastyk, "measures closeness to God: the history of this dimension is the account of how the present manifest situation evolved, or descended, from an original, pristine world of absolute unity."[5] The vertical dimension of the story explains how the knowledge in the text is revered as having descended from a faultless source, only to be consumed, digested (or interpreted), and disseminated by us, fallible human beings on earth who live day-to-day mostly along the horizontal dimension. Each of the medical narratives presented in this book combines these two dimensions to some extent. What is more, each narrative encapsulates what Wujastyk nicely describes as "a kind of *apologia*, and explanation of how something which was (past tense!) perfect, is now presented, brought into the present, in the blemished, mundane form of a textbook. It is an account of how knowledge which was once privileged is now commonly accessible."[6] The degree to which the medical narratives of Āyurveda were "commonly accessible" throughout Indian history until perhaps the decades just prior to British colonialism is often difficult to determine. Wujastyk's suggestion that these stories lay privilege on the origins and sources of knowledge of these texts—however mythic they may be—is useful to my investigation of the interplay between medicine and religion in Indian history. I would slightly nuance Wujastyk's reading to suggest that the information of these medical stories was always common knowledge and widely known. Such ubiquity of knowledge is what sets apart the narrative portions of the Sanskrit medical literature from the tradition's chart talk. Narrative medical explanations hence attend to the medically untrained community of patients, while at the same time they add social and moral weight to the medical compilers' rationalizations of disease and health. Without fail, the medical narratives of Āyurveda assign substantial weight to the actions of the gods and goddesses and demons that generally "give birth" to the diseases I discuss in the following chapters. That these figures are of a more pristine nature than humanity, and these stories shift back and forth across the vertical and horizontal dimensions of existence quite fluidly, suggests a tacit recognition by the medical compilers that disease and patienthood are endemic to the human condition (and after all, the stain of illness cannot stay in the heavens). But the process of becoming a patient, of acquiring disease, is one in which certain choices and social behaviors necessarily play a part.

This book is about medical storytelling and the socioreligious implications of particular illnesses that the compilers of India's Sanskrit medical literature saw fit to present narratively as unfolding over time, as opposed to depicting a body already infected, manifesting a certain disorder in need of treatment. By examining the beginnings, middles, and ends of narrative explanations for well- and ill-being in the classical literature of Āyurveda, I demonstrate that the compilers of this tradition meant to illustrate their decisions about the causes and effects of disease, as Rita Charon has put it, by "imposing plots on otherwise chaotic events."[7] The plots of the medical narratives that occur in the Indian medical literature tackle and systematize various strands of cultural discourse—social, ethical, and political—into coherent stories of patients' implicit health, falls into infirmity, and returns to health. Through the use of narratives, the compilers of the medical literature tackle both practical and ethical issues inherent to the human condition in the manner of Aristotle's "practical rationality," which seeks to establish the proper ends of human agency and the appropriate means for reaching them.[8] Practical rationality in the Aristotelian sense benefits humankind by effecting *eudaimonia*, the state of being well or human flourishing. In Cheryl Mattingly's ethnography of occupational therapists, Aristotelian practical rationality is at the heart of medical storytelling. Aristotle, she wrote, "associated the expert practical actor with a virtuous actor, one who is able to correctly see how to act in a given situation. Even apparently simple actions require an expertise that is more like acquired wisdom (what Aristotle called 'intelligence') than mere competence, because they require the actor to ascertain what the right action should be in a given case."[9] Mattingly discovered that storytelling in the biomedical setting serves the purpose of processing lived human experience and understanding practical activity in one's environment. Fully developed narratives about the body in Āyurveda similarly establish definitions and programs for attaining equally grand and oftentimes ethical goals: health (*ārogya, svāsthya*), long life (*āyus*), and good conduct (*sadvṛtti*). In addition to physiologic and mental health matters, they therefore address issues such as social relationships, sexual politics, and religion. The basic difference between the clinical reasoning of ayurvedic chart talk and narrative reasoning is this: whereas clinical reasoning provides the "is" of disease—for example, illness X is this and it can be cured in such and such a manner—narrative reasoning tends to attribute an agentive "ought" to the origins of disease—for example, illness X affects this person and not that person, because this person ought to have acted in a certain way but chose not to. With an "ought" ascribed to illness, Sanskrit medical narratives foreground social relations that the tradition's compilers perceived to produce disease and bodily dysfunction. Consequently, medical maladies may be understood and cured only by addressing the synthesis of social, moral, and physical agency in the life of a patient.

The Sanskrit medical stories constitute a specific tradition within Āyurevda that posits connections between gestures-actions-thoughts and health-illness and explains how and why people become patients in ways that are considered neither in biomedical pedagogy nor (with few exceptions) in recent scholarship on biomedical practice. The stories discussed in this book, which foreground the social forces underlying disease, as well as the hermeneutical methods I apply to them, can extend and enrich the methodological scope of scholarship in the medical humanities in America over the last few decades, which has tended to see social relations as having a "phantom objectivity," as Michael Taussig put it, following György Lukács, that obfuscates the social forces undergirding disease.[10] The stories of Āyurveda warrant careful inquiry into their function and placement within the tradition. Yet, they are often blatantly disregarded by practitioners and scholars of Āyurveda. During periods of fieldwork in South India in 2003–05, 2008, and 2011 at Government Ayurvedic Colleges, I frequently met students and practitioners of Āyurveda who dismissed the narrative tradition in the Sanskrit texts out of hand as useless to their work. There is no question, as I demonstrate in the chapters on fever, miscarriage, and the king's disease, that the stories in the ayurvedic sources have long and complex lives in religious literature (*Atharvaveda, Mahābhārata,* Purāṇas), moral-political-legal science (*dharmaśāstra*), and the science of statecraft (*arthśāstra*) that well exceed the medical context. The stories are there, however, and their removal or disavowal by modern practitioners has the same result of discounting the social factors that contribute to the causes and cures of disease that Taussig observed in studies of biomedicine among medical anthropologists in the United States in the early and mid-twentieth century.

People who read the medical literature of India in Sanskrit and in translation, such as medical practitioners, scholars, and those casually interested in alternative medicine, generally do not know that the medical literature of Āyurveda played an important role in the production of knowledge about religion, philosophy, and literature in Indian history. However small the physical size of the contribution of the medical narrative texts may be in comparison to the standard (i.e., non-narrative) medical discourse, without a study of these stories we are deprived of a valuable body of literature that rounds out our understanding of the history of both medicine and religions in India. And while the sheer number of medical stories in the medical literature may be small, the actual breadth of the medical literature covered by the primary narrative cycles (not to mention the magnum opus of Ānandarāyamakhin, the *Jīvānandanam,* which I cover in Chapter 6) that I introduce in this book is great. No less than eight Sanskrit medical compendia, and numerous non-medical sources, enter my discussion about the forms and functions of narrative in Indian medical history and literature. Much of the medical material, moreover, has never been presented in English.

At a metalevel, the medical narratives presented in this book can add substantially to cross-cultural and cross-disciplinary conversations about the ethics of illness in general, that is, the costs of being sick for oneself and society; medical representation and management of the human body; and the consequences of this management for the recipients of health care, the patients. In the Sanskrit literature of classical Āyurveda, representing and managing the body through storytelling is a highly pedagogical enterprise about how to use and not to use the body. The morals of these stories are in effect somatic lessons for patients, the tradition's designated "diseased ones" (*rogins*). The central aim of each medical narrative in classical Āyurveda is to assign responsibility for the condition of a body, to make a certain type of person perceived negatively—the sexual deviant, the ritual shirker, the egocentric, and so on—accountable for the health or illness of a body under discussion in the text. My contributions to this conversation in the South Asian context are novel. At present there is a dearth of scholarship on the medical patient in the South Asian context. Analyses of ayurvedic physicians and their regimens in premodern India are available, such as P. V. Sharma's *Rogī-parīkṣa-vidhi,* Kenneth Zysk's *Asceticism and Healing in Ancient India,* and Dagmar Wujastyk's *Well-Mannered Medicine.* While they add to our understanding of the doctor-patient relationship in the history of Āyurveda, they tend to emphasize the physician and the medical cohort more than the ayurvedic patient and patienthood. Excellent theoretical and ethnographic work has been done on patienthood in the biomedical contexts of the United States and Europe in recent decades, and I draw on this scholarship at times in this book to elucidate the figure of the patient in premodern South Asia. To discover the challenges and advantages of understanding the patient in the Indian medical literature for audiences working outside the small field of Indian medical history, my treatment of scholarship on patienthood and illness narratives outside of South Asia in Chapter 7 will be useful.

The patient in Āyurveda's narratives, who is portrayed either as human or, by mythic analogy, as divine, gets typecast as the good seed gone bad: the patient's material health suffers on account of his or her reprehensible social and religious actions. This image contrasts dramatically with the standard image of the patient in the non-narrative parts of Āyurveda, who is almost invariably a human being reducible to his or her diseased body. In the medical narratives, the patient's body is not passive and without experience but relational and active. In this way, Āyurveda's narratives effectively trace the onset of biophysical infirmity to the moral actions and social associations of patients. They mix medical data with normative points of view on social and religious agency so that morality and physiology become indivisible. The moral component of medical discourse connects personal motivation, social expectations, and religious practice to the determination of well-being. The links developed between socioreligious behavior and biophysical deterioration create an elaborate ontological pathology that the compilers of the ayurvedic tradition explored and supported through theoretical articulations of the self (*ātman*) and its relation to the material body (*śarīra*).

Intended Audience

In what follows, I examine the nature of medical discourse in classical Indian medicine primarily through three elaborate narrative traditions in ayurvedic literature—on fever, on miscarriage, and on the so-called king's disease—and one extensive allegory—*The Joy of Life* (*Jīvānandanam*). Medical narratives surrounding these conditions consistently relate the message that religious practice, self-knowledge, and patterns of social relationships one way or another produce and influence the development of certain diseases and biophysical dysfunctions in the human body. Narrative in Āyurveda is therefore an important heuristic device for explaining the social sources of illness, positing a specific account of reality, and depicting visions of how people ought to live as social actors in that posited reality. Āyurveda's narratives are a distinctively medical type of socioreligious, or dharmic, discourse, that is concurrently descriptive and normative. Their very occurrence suggests that medicine in classical India was used sometimes as an instrument for socioreligious instruction and control.

The substance and issues taken up in this book are aimed at three general audiences: people interested in Indian medicine, people interested in the history of Indian religions, and people interested in religious forms of healing and the intersection of medicine, morality, and religion. The central contribution of this project is its examination of Sanskrit illness narratives as lenses through which to view the role of religion in the historical development and practice of Indian medicine. This research makes a vital contribution to this important cultural history. I offer an original hermeneutical method for reading ayurvedic renderings of the body as clinical topography and the patient as social agent. My theoretical approach to reading medical narratives complements current work in the discipline of medical anthropology, particularly concerning the association of medical discourse and socioreligious ethics and relationships of power among cultural institutions. I also present and analyze important and understudied texts that add depth to current trends in the history of religions and the history of medicine in India.

For readers interested in religious forms of healing and the intersection of medicine, morality, and religion, I have attempted to bring together and analyze several ways that narrative logic in South Asian religions has been adapted in the classical medical context to explain health and illness. In so doing, it is my hope that this study will bring attention to uniquely South Asian narrative forms that are used to structure contemporary clinical practice and to create experiences for patients within and outside the doctor–patient encounter.

Plan of the Book

The next chapter, Chapter 2, contains the histories, both factual and mythic, and contents of the Sanskrit sources I use most often in the book, the *Carakasaṃhitā* and the *Suśrutasaṃhitā*. Much of the medical information I introduce is not available in a single, concise, and unified narrative, but instead is treated in introductions to individual editions of the Sanskrit medical sources, which often are not in English. Or, of course, one may consult Meulenbeld's massive five-volume *A History of Indian Medical Literature* (hereafter *HIML*), which is unexcelled by any other single source published in the past half century, "not only for medical history, but for Indology as a whole."[11] So, for the sake of convenience I offer basic yet crucial information about the history of Āyurveda that will be useful to contextualize the production and contemporary use of the sources I employ here. I end Chapter 2 with a discussion of the various renderings of human anatomy in the classical ayurvedic sources and explain the general schemata the sources use to classify diseases, prognoses, and therapies.

In Chapters 3 and 4, I focus on the narrative cycles of fever and miscarriage, respectively; in Chapter 5, I examine medical narratives about the king's disease, and, in Chapter 6, I discuss Ānandarāyamakhin's allegory about King Life and King Disease, *The Joy of Life*. In each of these chapters I have three overarching aims. The first aim is largely philological. Looking at the sociolinguistic bases of the major terms used in the narratives of each disease, and tracing the histories of each disease and the literary traditions from which the medical narratives about them derive, I illustrate the ways in which the tradition's compilers adapted the stories and disease etiologies, all of which have variants in non-medical sources, to the medical context. The second aim of the these four chapters is to explain the relationship between disease and medical patient in each narrative, while highlighting the associations drawn in the stories between society, religion, and the origin and development of disease. My third aim is to probe the contextualization of the patient in the narratives of fever, miscarriage, and the king's disease to gather information about the potential consequences of the stories' somatic lessons to be gleaned about physical comportment and living in the world as a healthy person.

In the conclusion, Chapter 7, I discuss the nature and function of narrative discourse in Āyurveda in particular and, more generally, in the medical context of the doctor–patient exchange in South Asia. To this end, I examine the ways in which narratives can function as vehicles for religious and social instruction in the medical context, and I conclude by focusing on the ideation and representation of the patient in Āyurveda. In view of the medical narratives and seven-act allegory I consider in Chapters 3 through 6, I mark out some of the general features of the ayurvedic patient in both the narrative and non-narrative medical discourse of the Sanskrit sources, and I query the theoretical and practical functions of the patient in Āyurveda and South Asia.

Chapter 2

The Patient's Body in Indian Medical Literature

The Sanskrit word *āyurveda* means "knowledge for long life." This translation reveals the objective (longevity), the means for achieving that objective (knowledge), and the breadth of coverage (life) of the medical system it so names: Āyurveda. Nothing less than the life of the human organism—a four-part aggregate composed of body, sense organs, mind, and self—is the subject of Āyurveda's professed knowledge.[1] In short, agreement among these four parts of human life generates health, whereas discord among them generates illness. Not every ayurvedic treatise tries to address the entirety of human life, however, or even the entirety of the human organism. Some specialize, some generalize, and others do a little of both. Methods of inquiry and analysis also differ, and there is an underlying debate in the medical sources concerning prognostic aptitude among ayurvedic physicians, known as vaidyas.[2] Even though the methods of investigation and analysis for the vaidya vary from one classical treatise to the next, the subject of the vaidya's enquiry—the body of the patient—is a constant point of reference throughout the medical literature.

Despite the ubiquity of the physical human body in the classical medical literature, the patient to whom each analyzed body belongs is an elusive and frequently hard-to-define feature within Āyurveda. A recurring theme throughout this book is that the patient is at once difficult to characterize yet indispensible in the classical ayurvedic corpus. The standard medical term for "patient" in Sanskrit is *rogin*, though *vyādhita* and *ātura* are also used with some regularity. All three of these terms are adjectives the compilers of Āyurveda's classical sources used nominally to mean "diseased or sick person." One classical source lists the patient as the fourth essential pillar of ayurvedic medicine, following the vaidya, medicine, and the attendant (sometimes translated as "nurse").[3] Yet, unlike Āyurveda's other two human foundations, the vaidya and the attendant, who actively administer medicine and medical knowledge, the patient routinely undergoes a near complete corporealization. That is, patients in the ayurvedic sources are systematically depicted as instruments, or mechanisms that are known and classified according to the flaws of their bodies. In reading the Sanskrit texts it is often difficult to know if the patient is a pronominal "who/m" or "what." Is the patient, in other words, a relational person? Or is the patient reducible to his or her body, a socially isolable thing? Surely the physiologically ill and biomechanically dysfunctional patients of ayurvedic literature are imagined to be and depicted as real people. They have specific genders, ages, and sometimes social standings as well (such as class and caste, *varṇa* and *jāti*). In the greater portion of every Sanskrit medical source, however, patients are represented as anonymous, generally static bodies, rather than, like the vaidya and attendant, formative subjects within the ayurvedic system. Their representations are determined by the medical system rather than, like the vaidya and the attendant, formative subjects within the system. Because of the continual focus on their somatic façades and internal functioning, patients in the classical sources usually are not active social actors with complex social positions and relationships that affect their physical and mental well-being. It is helpful to phrase the conception of the patient in the medical literature in grammatical terms, for the texts themselves use verbal language exclusively (that is, sans illustrations) to depict the human body and therefore the patient. The patient, the "diseased one," is almost always a pronominal "what" rather than an acting nominative "who" or even a passively accusative "whom." This is especially clear in descriptions of the patient as a "site of work to be done" (*kāryadeśa*) and the regular analogizing of patients' bodies with agricultural terrain.[4] This may also point to an agricultural source of Indian medicine, a kind of "folk medicine." Such verbal sketches unveil the degree to which the patient is at once a crucial theoretical and practical contrivance in the ayurvedic design. The patient is, I argue throughout this book, a workable object for medical forensics in classical Indian medicine and the fundamental practical site on which to apply the tradition's knowledge for long life.

That the hub of India's classical medical system could be any human body, rather than a specific body tied to a uniquely individual life with a detailed history, is hardly surprising. By way of illustration, take the famous medical textbook of 1858 widely used in biomedical schools, *Gray's Anatomy*.[5] Most people know that this book is not about the anatomy of a person named Gray. The Gray of the title refers to the work's author, the anatomist Henry Gray. For purposes of educating physicians to prepare for clinical medicine, it is unnecessary for the bodies of prototypical patients to be anything more than material entities that exhibit symptoms and pathologies with tendencies to react in one way or another when they are under the influence of certain drugs and therapies. How, then, do we understand and interpret the Sanskrit medical sources that describe patients as socially engaged and emotional human beings, people who are clearly more than mere mechanistic or material entities? Moreover, how do we properly read the specific passages in the medical compendia that typically occur in narrative form, given that the social and ethical activity of the patients in these stories is at the very heart of the compendia's etiologies for human health and illness? To do this, a special hermeneutics of medical discourse is needed. The narratives of Āyurveda attest to the significance of social syntax in medical explanation. Pathology trumps nosology in these stories, and in so doing they challenge some of the bases of the very scientific literature they inhabit. In the last half century, few people have advanced the hermeneutics of medical discourse more than Michel Foucault. His careful study of the origins of the medical clinic in particular is helpful to the present study. For Foucault, in the idiom of the clinic, "one is dealing with diseases that happen to be afflicting this or that patient: what is present is the disease itself, in the body that is appropriate to it, which is not that of the patient, but that of its truth."[6] The patient is merely a vessel for the disease, which is the medical example physicians aspire to know and name. The work of clinical physicians is to present texts that verify their a priori arrived at truths about disease, while the patient is epiphenomenal.

In the narratives of Indian medical literature that present the process of becoming ill, which naturally ends in the state of patienthood, we find a counterview of the clinical gaze that Foucault chronicled. The role of the physicians who adapted the stories of Āyurveda for the medical context appears not to be one of mere naming and nosological indexing that characterizes the clinical demonstration in Foucault's terms, or what I describe in the Introduction as the chart talk of the Sanskrit sources. The medical narrative opens up a space in which to examine the patient thoroughly and contextually. By presenting a story of a person's procession into patienthood, it seeks to arrive at the truth of sickness and health not by showing or demonstrating a set of presupposed truths but by discovering the experience of illness through an examination of the social and cultural factors that contribute to well-being and health.[7] When the authors of the Sanskrit medical sources present stories about patients and their activities, we learn four critical things about the nature of the patient in Āyurveda that is not apparent elsewhere in the literature. First, patients have lives through which they navigate by means of their physical bodies. Second, patients are complex human beings whose social competence and standing in the world amounts to the embodiment of the medical tradition's ideas about sickness and health. Third, in the course of their lives, patients' bodies undergo physical changes from ostensible states of health to ostensible states of sickness. And fourth, the ways in which patients choose to navigate their lives, engaging in and withdrawing from any number of activities and relationships, will determine whether or not they can regain better health after having fallen ill. Narrative discourse, or storytelling, is the primary means in the Sanskrit medical sources to illustrate the somatic transformation from healthfulness to illness as well as, critically, the implications of this transformation for living in the world. In the tradition's chart talk discussions of health and illness in anonymous, inert, and theorized bodies of patients, such sweeping life processes are entirely unexpressed.

In ayurvedic literature there are significant junctures where the medical authors' use of narrative discourse occludes more common methods of biophysiologic inquiry in favor of stories in which etiologies of diseases are linked to activities of deities and demons, legendary sages, and extraordinary human beings. Many of these narratives properly belong to the genre of mythology. For the moment, it suffices to say that the medical narratives of classical Indian medicine are conspicuous in the medical literary context because they do not, like most accounts of the human body in the literature, catalogue the minutiae of the human body's structure and physiologic functioning to explain matters of health and illness. The pathologies and prescriptions of the medical narratives tend to be more axiological and ontological than biophysical, echoing the patient perspectives of illness as morally laden and socially contingent in Deborah Lupton's historiography of biomedicine, so that the experience of being ill moves beyond mere physical suffering and entails notions of personal worth and sense of self.[8] Illnesses are contextualized outside of the material body in these stories, and they are viewed as products of the social spaces and patterns of relationships that exist between, rather than inside of, human bodies. To differentiate and contextualize the narrativization of the body, which is the focus of the following four chapters, from a characteristic chart talk–type dissertation on the body and disease in Indian medical literature, it is helpful to look at how bodies and diseases are classified and understood to operate in the classical Sanskrit sources.

Medical Context and Organization

The kind of knowledge useful to ensure long life—that is, the specific data, methods, and values that characterize the general concerns of Āyurveda—pertains primarily to the superintendence of the human body.[9] The primary resources for medical knowledge in India in the early centuries of the Common Era about health and illness in the human body are the Sanskrit compendia of Āyurveda. The knowledge systems that shape the Sanskrit sources are highly reticulated. They often incorporate elements of earlier and coeval Indian intellectual traditions, including philosophical logic (Nyāya), the science of particularities (Vaiśeṣika), social-legal-religious ethics (Dharmaśāstra), astronomy (Jyotiṣa), philosophical cosmology (Sāṃkhya), and Buddhism.[10] But like many types of Sanskrit literature, the literature of Āyurveda also has its own mythological account of its knowledge formation and pedigree.

For example, the *Suśrutasaṃhitā* explains that the god Brahmā composed the medical knowledge that would become classical Āyurveda. Originally, his collection of data consisted of 100,000 verses (*ślokas*), which was spread over 1,000 chapters. But Brahmā quickly discovered that humans did not live long enough, not to mention that they lacked the intelligence, to memorize so many verses. So he divided his medical teachings into eight divisions, or "adjunct parts" (*aṅgas*), to make this knowledge easier for humanity to learn and remember. The eight divisions are:

1. internal medicine (*kāyacikitsā*)
2. ear-, nose-, and throat-related medicine (*śālākya*)
3. surgery (*śalya*)
4. poison treatment or toxicology (*viṣacikitsā* or *agadatantra*)
5. demonology (*bhūtavidyā*)
6. embryological-, obstetric-, and pediatric-related medicine (*kaumārabhṛtya*)

7. rejuvenation therapy (*rasāyana*)
8. sexual enhancement (*vājīkaraṇa*—literally, "making like a stallion")

Every medical text positions the eight divisions differently, so that each text draws attention to the importance of one division over the others depending on the work's general focus or specialization. So, for example, the medical work specializing in surgery, the *Suśrutasaṃhitā*, declares *śalya* to be the foremost branch of ayurvedic medicine, whereas the work focusing on embryology, obstetrics, and pediatrics, the *Kāśyapasaṃhitā*, gives *kaumārabhṛtya* pride of place among the eight. It is, however, important to note that to call these eight types of medicine divisions or adjunct parts is somewhat misleading. The Sanskrit sources are not typically divided into sections according to these divisions. Instead, one or more of the eight foci of Āyurveda are usually interspersed throughout a work's various theoretical and methodological "sections" (*sthānas*), which regularly include some, if not all, of the following: an initial overview (*sūtrasthāna*); a section on pathology (*nidānasthāna*); a section on measurements (*vimānasthāna*); a section on the body (*śārīrashtāna*); a section on the sense organs (*indriyasthāna*); a section on internal medicine (*cikitsāsthāna*); a section on ritual precepts (*kalpasthāna*); and a section on efficacious treatment (*siddhisthāna*). Some of the classical sources also have an appendix, or supplementary section (*uttaratantra* or *uttarasthāna*). The body is the lodestone of each of these sections, yet the ways in which the body is depicted from section to section in any one text, not to mention from text to text, is far from uniform.

Bodytalk I: Diseases, Prognoses, and Therapies

Several words in classical Indian medical literature designate the human body. The terms *śarīra, deha, tanus, kāya,* and *vapus* are the words most commonly used to mean "body." Occasionally the terms *gātra* and *aṅga,* both of which can mean "adjunct part" or "component" (Sanskrit lexicographers in the eighteenth-nineteenth centuries traditionally translated these words as "limb" or "member"), synecdochically signify the entire physical body as well. The philosophically and religiously important and multilayered word *ātman,* usually translated in English as "self," referring to the immaterial personal principle that moves from lifeform to lifeform in the cycle of rebirth and redeath, sometimes also indicates the physical body in the classical sources. The variety of names deployed to denote the human body reflects the highly synonymic nature of the Sanskrit language, rather than, for example, alternative means, designated by each term (*śarīra, deha, tanus,* and so on), for applying ayurvedic knowledge in pursuit of long life.

Many of the Sanskrit medical sources locate their bodytalk in a specified section on the body (*śārīrasthāna*), though this does not hold true across the entire ayurvedic corpus. The compendia of Caraka, Suśruta, Bhela, and Kaśyapa, and the two works attributed to Vāgbhaṭa, the *Aṣṭāṅgahṛdayasaṃhitā* and the *Aṣṭāṅgasaṃgrahasaṃhitā*, have sections on the body. There is little uniformity across these body sections, however. Hence there is not a consistent representation of the minutiae of the human body from one source to the next. The most extensive description and analysis of the body occurs in the text largely devoted to the science of surgery, the *Suśrutasaṃhitā*.[11] The details of the diverse anatomical rendering in Āyurveda are rather extensive, so I will not rehearse all of discrepancies here but, by way of explanation, point to just a few of them. The *Carakasaṃhitā* and the *Bhelasaṃhitā* each identifies six layers of skin (*tvac*), whereas the *Suśrutasaṃhitā* identifies seven.[12] The *Carakasaṃhitā, Bhelasaṃhitā,* and *Kāśyapasaṃhitā* calculate the number of bones (*asthi*s) in the human body, including teeth and nails, at 360, where the *Suśrutasaṃhitā* counts 300.[13] The *Carakasaṃhitā, Suśrutasaṃhitā, Aṣṭāṅgahṛdayasaṃhitā,* and *Aṣṭāṅgasaṃgrahasaṃhitā* state that the human body has 900 ligaments (*snāyu*s), whereas the *Bhelasaṃhitā* simply states that there are ligaments in the body without indicating a specific number.[14] The number of arterial vessels or veins—literally "pipes" or "tubes" inside the body (*dhamanī*s)—total 200 in both the *Carakasaṃhitā* and *Kāśyapasaṃhitā*. Yet there are considerably fewer, just 24, in the *Suśrutasaṃhitā, Aṣṭāṅgahṛdayasaṃhitā,* and *Aṣṭāṅgasaṃgrahasaṃhitā*.[15] And this list could go on and on.

How do we account for such discrepancies in somatic knowledge in the classical medical sources? One certain reason for the divergence of understanding stems from the lengthy durations of time over which the Sanskrit medical sources were composed and compiled, sometimes spanning centuries. People from different generations, with different knowledge of and access to the human body, redacted, emended, and added to these works. The diversity of authorship within a specific text's genealogy—including composers, redactors, and commentators—may account for some of the anatomical inconsistencies across the ayurvedic corpus. Another reason may have to do with the fact that, apart from physicians trained in the surgical branch of medicine, the details of which are preserved in the *Suśrutasaṃhitā*, among classical Indian physicians there appears to have been a glut of inexperience in the practice of dissection, which is crucial to accurate anatomical explanation.[16] Even so, although the surgical skills of the physicians who compiled and were trained according to the *Suśrutasaṃhitā* were evidently far more advanced than those of the compilers and students of the other classical compendia, the accuracy of their conceptions of the human body should be viewed with the knowledge that they, like their contemporaries in classical India, had limited access to human bodies for dissection. We read in the text itself that even physicians associated with the *Suśrutasaṃhitā* trained on nonhuman objects and bodies, such as animal carcasses, gourds, and the hollow trunks of plants to prepare for surgery on humans. Kenneth Zysk has also demonstrated that the use of nonhuman bodies and objects as preparatory models for human surgery and dissection speaks to another potential reason for the frequently conflicting portraits of the body in the ayurvedic sources: namely, prevailing concerns with ritual purity and pollution in classical Hindu societies, for anxiety over ritual purity could have deterred physicians from engaging in dissection because the practice naturally involved contact with polluting substances, such as blood, bile, mucus membrane, and the like.[17]

Despite inconsistencies in language concerning the intricacies of the body, there are some general classificatory schemata that the classical sources maintain, which reveal a coherent systematization of knowledge about the body that extends across the literature. Disease classification is a good example. Diseases in Āyurveda typically assail the body, the mind, or the sense organs.[18] The eleventh-century commentator, Cakrapāṇidatta, cites the following examples of diseases that affect, respectively, the body, mind, and sense organs: a tumor, adherence to untruths, and partial blindness (or cataracts).[19] Types of diseases are further classified according to a two-, three-, or fourfold system. In the *Aṣṭāṅgahṛdayasaṃhitā*, we find a twofold classification of internal (*nija*) and invasive (*āgantu*) diseases.[20] The *Carakasaṃhitā* identifies three types of disease: internal, invasive, and mental (*mānasa*).[21] The *Suśrutasaṃhitā* recognizes four types: invasive, mental, bodily, and natural (*svābhāvika*).[22] Internal diseases in the *Carakasaṃhitā* and *Aṣṭāṅgahṛdayasaṃhitā* generally align with so-called bodily diseases in the *Suśrutasaṃhitā*. These are generally attributable to the morbidity of a body's humors and a person's diet. Invasive diseases in all three works are attributable to influences outside the body, such as demons, gods, poisons, wind, and combat; a person's actions, or *karmans*, are also frequently said to produce invasive diseases. Mental diseases in the

Carakasaṃhitā are said to arise from not getting what one wants in life or, conversely, getting what one does not want. In the *Suśrutasaṃhitā*, mental diseases are produced by emotional temperaments like anger, grief, fear, pleasure, lust, and so forth. The natural category of disease in the *Suśrutasaṃhitā* includes things that are physiologically given with every human body, such as hunger, thirst, old age, and death.

Central to the ayurvedic conception of the actively living human body, that is, a body engaged with the world of objects and people, are the last of the three targets of disease, the sense organs. In Sanskrit, the term for a sense organ is *indriya*. The function of a body's *indriya*s is to ascertain and process knowledge (*jñānendriya*). An *indriya* is not an internal bodily mechanism in the biomedical sense of the word "organ," however. In fact, in Āyurveda the body's organs, such as the stomach or liver, appear by the rather vague label of "containers" (*āśaya*s). Dominik Wujastyk has shown that the organs of the human body are not understood to operate in Āyurveda in the same way they are understood and described to operate in biomedical discourse—as industrious mechanisms that digest food, churn out nutrients, remove toxins from the blood, and so forth.[23] Because of the radical difference between the body's organs in Āyurveda and biomedicine, Francis Zimmerman has suggested that classical Āyurveda does not have a bona fide anatomy at all, in the Western sense of the term anatomy. Sanskrit medical literature is not as concerned as biomedicine with anatomy and substance, in Zimmerman's view, but instead tends to focus on pathology and process.[24] This is a very provocative position, to which I return at the end of this chapter. The classical ayurvedic conception of the sense organs likely comes from the Vedic use of the word *indriya* as "power" or "force" (usually associated with the god Indra). In Sanskrit medical literature, *indriya* signifies a force or power of the body, such as the sense faculties and powers of perception. The classical medical sources characteristically use the term *indriya* to address questions of perception. The *indriya*s are "organs" insofar as they are means, forces, or modi operandi that enable a person to know and interact with the world. Yet the *indriya*s are not organs in the same way that biomedical anatomy texts represent the heart, liver, and eyes. The *indriya*s are not visible; their existence is inferable as being present in the ears, nose, eyes, tongue, and skin. People know the *indriya*s are present and working properly because they pick up specific auditory, olfactory, visual, tasteable, and tactile objects that are principally associated with them (as shown in Figure 1).

In Āyurveda the body's containers (*āśaya*s) are somewhat like the organs in characteristic biomedicine inasmuch as these containers

Sense Organs (*indriyas*)	**Sense Objects** (*arthas*)	**Containers** (*āśayas*)
Through the means of ...	... one encounters ...	... in/on the ...
hearing	sounds	ears
smell	scents	nose
sight	visual images	eyes
taste	tastes	tongue
touch	textures	skin

Figure 1. Sense Organs in Classical Āyurveda

hold and circulate fluids, the humors, and blood throughout the body. In addition to processing perceptual knowledge, these containers are linked to the organs of bodily activity. The body's "action organs" (*karmendriyas*), such as the larynx, genitals, feet, anus, and hands, house the sense organs, without which, in turn, the hands could not apprehend, the feet could not ambulate, the eyes could not see, and so on.

Disease prognosis is another area in which the classical medical sources exhibit a common organization. Diseases generally fall within the following threefold classification: curable (*sādhya*), treatable but not curable (*yāpya*), and incurable (*asādhya*).[25] The *Carakasaṃhitā* and *Aṣṭāṅgahṛdayasaṃhitā* further distinguish two types of curable diseases: diseases that are easily curable (*sukhasādhya*) and those that are difficult to cure (*kṛcchrasādhya*). Likewise for the incurable, there are two types: those that may be palliated (*syādyāpya*) and those that are irreversible (*anupakramayāpya*).[26] The *Carakasaṃhitā* adds that physicians who cannot properly distinguish between the three types of disease will lose their money, knowledge, and fame, and will incur a bad reputation.[27] Accordingly, the classical sources repeatedly advise physicians and their students to avoid taking on patients with incurable diseases.[28]

According to the *Carakasaṃhitā*, there are three general types of remedial plant-based therapy (*oṣadhi*) in Āyurveda. One involves the gods and goddesses, another entails the physician's reasoning skills during the evaluation of a patient, and the last one concerns the health of the mind.[29] In the following chapters, I am mainly concerned with the kind of medical care that involves divine influences (*daiva*). Among other things, the kind of medicine that involves deities includes recitation of mantras, religious austerities, ritual practice, sacrifice, deity worship, and pilgrimage. These therapies are regularly linked to diseases ostensibly stemming from the ways in which people comport themselves in society, and they are justified according to the worldviews and religious ideologies of the authors who describe them. To articulate such therapies and diseases, standard chart talk is insufficient. Narrative discourse is essential to elaborate the perceived connection between behavior, social and religious axiology, and disease. Historians of Indian medicine have paid scant attention to the narrative cycles of the classical Sanskrit medical literature, often quickly dismissing these sections in the medical sources as late, religious (or brahminical) interpolations in an imaginary Ur-science of ancient India. Such an argument is difficult to prove on the basis of the extant literature. And more importantly, it also fails to note the cultural and historical symbiosis of religion, medicine, and politics illustrated in the medical literature. The compilers and purveyors of the ayurvedic classics were important commentators on and producers of classical Indian religious discourse, ritual practice, and social construction. As I show in the chapters on fever, miscarriage, and the king's disease, the narratives in the medical sources were not produced exclusively in a medical or scientific context. The authors of the medical sources effectively recycled these narratives from other Sanskrit corpora, touching on subjects such as philosophy, religion and statecraft, and they adapted them to specific medical agendas. The reuse and adaptation of stories from non-medical cultural domains has the bold effect of introducing commentary on ethical and aesthetic value into the medical program. In particular, these stories help us to understand how the history of Indian religions has informed the history of Indian medicine. They also present an as-yet untapped perspective on, and Sanskrit-based interpretation of, the history of religions in India.

The narratives of Āyurveda are rich documents of Indian cultural history. Through the medium of storytelling, they bring together elements from social domains that today we typically pigeonhole as autonomous institutions from medicine, religion, and politics. They thus provide a valuable historical service by expanding the horizons of our reading of both medical and religious histories in India as multifaceted and complex literary cultures. That said, while mining the narratives of Āyurveda for their cultural insights, we would be wrong to "de-medicalize" them and overlook their intended design as psychosomatically efficacious tools. A hermeneutics of medical discourse in the case of the Sanskrit medical sources requires that attention paid to intertextual and intercultural relationships within the narratives neither overshadows nor diminishes the important contribution of these stories to somatic treatment in classical Āyurveda. They belong to a type of therapy the *Kāśyapasaṃhitā* identifies as medicine that uses nonpharmaceutical therapies (*anauṣadha*, also simply called "curing," *bheṣaja*), which the text pairs with medicine that uses pharmaceutical therapies (*auṣadha*).[30] The *Carakasaṃhitā* classifies narrative medicine as therapy dependent on divine power (*daivāśrayauṣadha*) as well as medicine consisting of no material ingredients (*adravyabhūta*).[31] Narrative medicine evokes the older, Vedic therapies that involved mythic etiologies and fixed spells, rituals, and chants for healing. In his eleventh-century commentary on the *Carakasaṃhitā*, Cakrapāṇidatta explains that medicine dependent on divine influence can in fact eliminate human disease, but its efficacy ultimately comes from the power of the gods, not the physician or the patient.[32]

Bodytalk II: The Three Humors

A significant and consistent element of ayurvedic bodytalk across classical, medieval, and early-modern Sanskrit literature concerns the veritable mediators of health and disease in the body, the *doṣa*s, often translated as "humors." The idea of the body's three humors in Āyurveda is a potentially fruitful conceptual bridge to transition from the strict empiricism that predominates the classical medical literature to the multidimensional narrative discourses of the tradition's literature. As I stated in the Introduction, the standard chart talk of ayurvedic literature portrays the human body as entirely detachable from the life-trajectory of the person to whom it belongs. That said, the humoral theory suggests that within ayurvedic empirical doctrine a notion exists that posits the human body as a microcosmic homologue of an all-encompassing, macrocosmic materiality known as *prakṛti*. The expansive worldview intimated by the humoral theory effectively opens up space for multiple discourses within the medical system to address aspects of human culture apart from medicine and anatomy, such as society, religion, environment, and politics.

Āyurveda identifies and explains illness using a logical system of pathobiology and applies therapeutics according to theoretical models. Among them, the foremost is the doctrine of the three doṣas (*tridoṣavidyā*): wind (*vāta*), bile (*pitta*), and phlegm (*kapha* or *śleṣman*).[33] Each humor has a natural seat in the body. Wind predominates in the pelvic region, bile in the abdomen, and phlegm in the chest. Yet the humors are constantly active and always intermingling with the body's seven fundamental substances (*dhātus*): chyle, blood, flesh, fat, bone, marrow, and semen. They also interact with the three categories of somatic waste products: urine, feces, and perspiration. Each humor has specific properties that determine its influence on the tissues of a body. For example, vāta is dry, cool, lightweight, and mobile; pitta is slightly oily, hot, lightweight, and prickly; and kapha is cold, slimy, heavy, and soft. To describe the breadth of humoral influence on the body, vāta, pitta, and kapha are further subdivided according to particular somatic location. For example, *prāṇa* is a type of the vāta-humor located in the head, chest, and neck; *pacaka* is a type of pitta-humor located in the duodenum and intestines; *kledaka* is a type of kapha-humor located in the chest and stomach; and so on. A significant difference between the body's humors, typically described as semifluid substances, and other somatic elements like blood, bones, and tendons is that the humors are said to be the body's primary pathogenic arbiters and regulators of health.[34] An excess or deficiency of one humor or an unnatural combination of humors in any area of the body is said to generate disease.

The source of Āyurveda's classical doctrine of the three humors is unknown. Hartmut Scharfe suggested that humoral theory in the compendia of Caraka, Suśruta, and Vāgbhaṭa developed on the basis of or alongside Buddhist canonical sources, and Kenneth Zysk's work on healing in ancient Indian Buddhist monasteries supports this claim.[35] Irrespective of the source, it is clear that ayurvedic humoral theory remains relatively unchanged from source to source in the Sanskrit literature. The Sanskrit word translated here as "humor" is *doṣa*, and its most basic meaning is "fault" or "taint." The earliest layer of Indian medical literature, found in the *Carakasaṃhitā* and the Buddhist Pali Canon, portrayed bile and phlegm in a neutral fashion. They were purely somatic elements, not thought to be negative or faults of any kind. Only later, with the *Suśrutasaṃhitā* and thereafter, do we find all three humors carrying the connotation of taint and fault when they are found to be in excess or deficient in certain areas of the body.[36] Clearly integral to the physiology of individual bodies, the humors also play a grander conceptual role in Āyurveda. They contribute to a worldview in which individual human bodies essentially converge with other bodies and, ultimately, with the cosmos by virtue of their shared material structure and constitutions. To fully understand the role of the humors in this regard, we need to look at ideas about the placement of humankind in the cosmos in both medical and nonmedical Sanskrit literature and then consider parallel ideas in the philosophical system of Sāṃkhya.

The medical sage Ātreya Punarvasu commented on the coterminous relationship existing between the constitutions of the human body and the cosmos very directly:

> The individual is of the same measure as the universe. As much as there is elemental diversity in the universe, in equal measure there is elemental diversity in the individual. As much as there is elemental diversity in the individual, in equal measure there is elemental diversity in the universe.[37]

For Ātreya the human body was a cosmos in miniature, the microcosmic counterpart to a universal macrocosm. Ideas about the natures of the cosmos and the body in Āyurveda echo cosmological reckoning in the classical dualistic philosophy of Sāṃkhya, as Gerald Larson's work has suggested, while Antonella Comba's investigation of parallels in ayurvedic thought and classical Vaiśeṣika reveals apparent shared commonalities between these two traditions as well.[38] Both of these scholars have sensibly shied away from postulating a chronology of influence or suggesting that one tradition likely influenced the other on these issues. A lot of ink has been spilled regarding the transmission of knowledge and which tradition can rightly claim credit for creating an idea and influencing others concerning that idea. Such speculation has surrounded the relationship between Āyurveda and Sāṃkhya for some time, particularly on the subjects of cosmology and the link between matter and spirit. The development of the two traditions were relatively coeval in Indian history, and as far as I can determine, there is no evidence conclusive enough to suggest one way or the other that where commonalities exist between Sāṃkhya and Āyurveda on matters of cosmology, matter, and spirit the origins of the shared ideas can be shown to belong originally to one tradition or the other.

Generally speaking, classical ayurvedic bodytalk recognizes equivalencies among the material makeup of the universe and human bodies, including such things as the qualities thought to inhere in all worldly objects, an all-pervasive self (*ātman*), and the five great elements (*mahābhūtas*)—earth (*pṛthivī*), water (*āpaḥ*), fire (*tejas* or *agni*), wind (*vāyu*), and space or ether (*ākāśa*).[39] On the subject of the five great elements constituting the universe and humankind, the compilers of the *Carakasaṃhitā* described the macro–micro correspondences between universal environment and human body in this way: "Earth comprises the solid form of the human being. Water makes up the moisture. Fire is the heat. Wind makes the breath. Space constitutes the hollow parts. *Brahman* is the interior self."[40] The view of the body's five primary elements and basic constituents may be traced back to the *Garbha Upaniṣad* of Pippālada in the *Black Yajurveda*, which outlines the formation of the embryo from conception to full bodily development.[41] This short Upaniṣad offers a brief view of notions developed more elaborately in classical Āyurveda that the internal milieu of a person's body is understood to interact with, and to be influenced by, environments external to it like the biosphere, family, and society. This is a theme that recurs throughout the medical tradition, most forcefully and entertainingly in the allegory *The Joy of Life*, which I discuss in Chapter 6. The linkages of corresponding elements across inner somatic and outer social fields are said to be critical determinants in the health of both the individual body and the body's external environments.

In the classical Sāṃkhya tradition, everything in the universe is made up of two opposing ontological principles: a masculine principle, *puruṣa*, which is pure unchanging spirit or consciousness; and a feminine principle, *prakṛti*, which is non-conscious materiality. The Sanskrit word *prakṛti* literally means "nature" or "matter," and Īśvarakṛṣṇa's *Sāṃkhyakārikā* uses the term *prakṛti* primarily to refer to the material world.[42] The relationship between *prakṛti* and *puruṣa* closely resembles the relationship of the material body and self, or ātman, described in the Upaniṣads.[43] Just as the ātman is housed in and motivates the material body, though it is not affected by the body's diseases, in the Sāṃkhyan system *puruṣa* is entangled in the material world of *prakṛti* yet spared the travail of recurrent material appearance and deterioration. The two principles are codependent, however, and each serves to define the contours of the other. Hence Tracy Pintchman noted that *puruṣa*'s "presence is nevertheless a vital component [of the material world], for it is only in the presence of *puruṣa*, the principle of pure consciousness, that *prakṛti* can evolve."[44] All material phenomena come into existence on account of *prakṛti*, which through a series of stages transforms from a nebulous state into a precise state in which numerous different categories emerge and evolve. Throughout this evolution the phenomenal world is organized into twenty-five elements of reality called *tattva*s, the twenty-fourth and twenty-fifth of which are *prakṛti* and *puruṣa*, respectively. The first twenty-four *tattva*s constitute the stuff of worldly existence, which consists of amalgams of three primary qualities called guṇas—*sattva* (lucidity, goodness), *rajas* (energy, passion), and *tamas* (darkness, inertia). Only *puruṣa* is devoid of these qualities. All things, including the mental faculties (intellect, ego, and mind), are made up of a combination of the guṇas, so that every aspect of creation may be classified according to its guṇa-preponderance. As long as a person is unaware of his or her true spirit, he or she remains fettered to the changing states of *prakṛti*, in which the interaction and transformation of guṇas incessantly give rise to the gross matter of worldly existence. In due course, *prakṛti* also causes all worldly things to pass away.[45] Only by realizing that *prakṛti* is utterly distinct from one's real, spiritual self can one become free from the unending effects of one's actions, explained in the philosophical principle of cause and effect known as karma, which fuels the saṃsāric cycle of repeated births and deaths into and out of the gross material world.

The physicality, propensity to deteriorate, and relative classification of the guṇas in Sāṃkhya correspond, theoretically, to Āyurveda's three humors. Gerald Larson rejected as "simplistic and unconvincing" the view of Ḍalhaṇa, twelfth-century commentator on the *Suśrutasaṃhitā*, that Āyurveda's vāta, pitta, and kapha neatly match Sāṃkhya's *rajas, sattva,* and *tamas*. Larson is right that a simple one-to-one correlation between these two fundamental doctrines in Āyurveda and Sāṃkhya is hardly possible, because, as he says, "technically speaking, *vāta, pitta,* and *kapha* are tamasic manifestations since they emerge from the *mahābhūta*-s, which themselves are derived from the tamasic form of *ahaṁkāra,* namely, the five subtle elements or *tanmātra*-s."[46] Whereas we may dismiss Ḍalhaṇa's postulation on the grounds of direct, one-to-one equivalence between the two doctrines, as Larson does, we may also read the *Suśrutasaṃhitā*'s commentator with a bit more liberality in our interpretation. As Larson himself noted, in major portions of the *Suśrutasaṃhitā* there is a clear bias toward Sāṃkhya philosophy. This partiality very well could have swayed Ḍalhaṇa's perspective, causing him to see more associations between the two knowledge systems than indeed existed, encouraging his oversimplification, if not mischaracterization, of the guṇa-doctrine. Nonetheless, we can still reasonably speak about a few broad commonalities between the doṣa and guṇa doctrines. For example, just as in Sāṃkhya disequilibria among the guṇas of *prakṛti* undulate matter across the cosmic horizon, in Āyurveda, when the humors are irritated (*prakupita*) or in a state of irregularity (*vaiṣamya*), disease materializes in the body. The guṇas and the doṣas also serve a similar taxonomic function. According to Sāṃkhya, the entire material world may be classified according to the predominance of one of the three guṇas; correspondingly, the ayurvedic physician identifies specific bodily disorders and illnesses according to the predominance of one of the doṣas in certain locations in a patient's body. In substance, moreover, both Sāṃkhya and Āyurveda accept that the tissues of the body are derived from the five great elements that constitute the universe. Francis Zimmermann has convincingly shown that the very same doṣic elements circulating in our bodies are also "circulating underground, in the water, in the air . . . everywhere around us and within us." Yet, crucially, unlike the Sāṃkhyan principle of *prakṛti,* he continues, "they are also forces, powers which foment disorders, pathogenic principles between which the doctor must establish justice."[47] The disorders and pathogenic principles Zimmermann mentions establish a kind of ontological pathology in Āyurveda, which underlies the sociobiological nature of the tradition by implicating in the determination of health and disease, in addition to the doṣas, social and ecological influences in a patient's life. To establish "justice" in the patient, the ayurvedic physician uses the knowledge of the Sanskrit sources to calculate a regimen that cultivates both the ātman and body of the patient. What is good for the patient, ultimately, not only eases the patient's internal humoral flow, but it also dovetails a patient's somatic physiology and life experience within a stream of affinity existing among one's individual body, other human and nonhuman life-forms, and one's ecosystem.

The individual person in Āyurveda is therefore divided, shared, and held in common among a multitude of forces in a way that calls to mind McKim Marriott's proposal that the Indian Hindu conceives humans as "dividuals" rather than individuals. Every person, in other words, is understood to be continuously engaged with other people and the natural world through the transference of what Marriott called "substance codes" that flow through food and water, alms, air, and the like, from person to person, people to animals, and creatures to the earth and atmosphere.[48] Francis Zimmermann has suggested something very similar to Marriott's notion of "dividuality" concerning the cosmic breadth of Āyurveda: "Through his food, habitat, and bodily techniques, the living being is influenced, penetrated, immersed in the system of the humors, flavors, and qualities that makes up the atmosphere, the climate, the landscape in which he takes root."[49] In other words, bodies in poor health for one reason or another are environmentally and cosmically crooked: the microscopic physiology of the body is not compatible with the environmental, macroscopic physiology of the universe. When an ayurvedic physician treats a patient, therefore, he or she must attempt to reestablish the lost balance between the somatic microcosm of the patient and the universal macrocosm.[50]

Medical Storytelling

In the medical storytelling of Āyurveda, the patient typically gets typecast as a good seed gone bad, either as a human being or allegorically via mythic analogy, whose physical health suffers on account of one or more reprehensible social and religious actions that she or he has committed. This image contrasts dramatically with the standard image of the patient in Āyurveda as a human being reducible to his or her diseased or healthy body. In the medical narrative, consequently, the patient's body is not passive and without experience but relational and active. In this way, Āyurveda's narratives effectively trace the onset of physical infirmities to the socioethical relations of patients. They mix medical data with normative perspectives on social and religious agency so that, following Francis Zimmermann's observation on the influence of religion in Āyurveda, "moral sentiments become indissociable from physiological effects."[51] The integration of morality in medical discourse implicates personal motivation, social expectations, and religious practice in the tradition's determination of well-being. Connections made between socioreligious behavior and biophysical deterioration contribute to an elaborate ontological pathology that the compilers of the classical medical system explored through theoretical articulations of the unchanging and transmigrating ātman and its relation to the material body.

Striking a highly instructive assertion about Āyurveda's utility, the *Carakasaṃhitā* reflects a pervasive outlook in the literature that the medical system's knowledge for long life attends to both the physical body and the immaterial ātman: "Knowers of the Vedas thought knowledge of long life [i.e., Āyurveda] was the most meritorious. It will be said that it is good for humankind in both worlds [i.e., the present and the next]."[52] Dominik Wujastyk has incisively observed that this claim in the *Carakasaṃhitā* reveals a kind of self-awareness that Āyurveda is "twice as useful" as strictly religious knowledge, such as the knowledge found in the Vedas.[53] The general idea is that the ayurvedic knowledge system first of all instructs people on the means to achieve the vital goal of a long and healthy life so that, secondarily, people may achieve other important, nonmedical goals, such as the "three things" (*trivarga*), more commonly known as the first three of the four valid aims of human life in Hinduism: dharma, material prosperity (*artha*), and sexual satisfaction (*kāma*).[54] To this end, the literature of Āyurveda may be read as promoting an expressly medical method for cultivating both the body and the self, called *ātmahita*, which literally means "one's good," or, adjectivally, denotes something that is "favorable to oneself."[55] Doing and surrounding oneself with things that are favorable to one's self constitutes what I argue is a complex and distinctively medical approach to personal cultivation intended to enhance a person's refinement of his or her somatic health so as to be able to attend to his or her socioreligious responsibilities, which fall under the tremendously important and especially difficult to define principle of dharma. The ways a person attends to his or her dharma, the medical narratives of Āyurveda suggest, in due course bear directly on a person's present lifetime, the ātman's journey through saṃsāra, and the forms a person's future lives will take.

Āyurveda's medical narratives, insofar as they clearly report the utter fundamentality of the material body to one's health and religious pursuits, articulate in an easily digestible and everyday manner the process of personal cultivation. These stories would have been useful for the tradition's compilers to relate the idea of personal cultivation of one's body and self to their students as well as their patients, for the philosophical components of the *ātmahita* concept are often recondite and require tedious unpacking and intertextual referencing to put it into plain words. It is noteworthy that Āyurveda's narratives underscore the social and religious dimensions of caring for and cultivating one's self and physical body. In these stories human bodies thrive or deteriorate not because they are congenitally prone to biophysical failure or because they are suddenly exposed to physical trauma. Rather, the narratives recount events in the lives of healthy people, or, more precisely, fabulous and godly figures who incur biophysical illnesses because they behave in certain ways and have attitudes that lead them to pursue things and foster relationships the preparers of the medical literature perceived to be unacceptable in some way. Patienthood becomes tied to states of being in the world, all of which are potential—literally embryonic—in every human life. The quality of being and becoming a sick or diseased person, a rogin, must be understood as having both bodily and socioreligious causes.

A discursive means for producing meaning about the body and its use in society, the medical narrative presents Āyurveda's social and religious teachings on the body, or somatic lessons to be incorporated into a person's regimen to enjoy a long and healthy life. We know very little about the people who composed and arranged the Sanskrit literature of Āyurveda. Apart from a collection of legendary physicians and their most outstanding pupils within the two major medical lines of Ātreya and Dhanvantari (about which I say more below), the general medical practitioner of classical India who might have been trained with these texts rarely appears in the present study as anything more than an "author," a "compiler," and a "vaidya."

The physicians of this period and the compilers of this literature were undoubtedly men. The patient will emerge piecemeal from chapter to chapter, not in name but in form and function, as a living, breathing, and relational human being whose life story is captured in the texts in episodic portraits that typically showcase his or her errant behavior. Intertextual references to coeval and earlier Sanskrit works in which these stories, or versions of these stories, crop up help to fill in the "biographies" of the people who play the role of patient in Āyurveda. The fundamental meaning that the narratives of Āyurveda impart, I hope to show, is an appreciation for life (*āyus*). The sentiment that "there is no gift more special than the gift of life," as the *Carakasaṃhitā* declares, permeates the various medical, sociological, and religious meanings in the medical narratives of classical Āyurveda discussed in this book.[56]

The Sanskrit medical sources do not have illustrations or sketches of the human body, even if, as the text-historical studies of Indian anatomy that Hoernle, Zysk, and Yamashita each duly confirms, the body is entirely central to Āyurveda.[57] Nor do these sources supply any kind of tables or diagrams that chart the bio-philosophical homologies between the physical universe, social order, and human body or provide diagrams to explain the malignant influence of omens and ghosts on a physical body to which the texts sometimes refer.[58] Whereas illustrations of course are not required to develop a thorough understanding of the human body in a medical knowledge system, this limits the present study to an examination of the ways in which the compilers of the Sanskrit medial sources used language to express information about the body. To grasp the range of abilities and utter indispensability of the body to the institution, literature, and practice of Āyurveda, it is essential to look not only at the presentation of the body's physical framework and internal functioning in the literature, but also at the social body in the narratives of the tradition. The stories I examine in the following chapters are taken from numerous Sanskrit sources, but four works in particular are central: the *Carakasaṃhitā*, *Suśrutasaṃhitā*, *Kāśyapasaṃhitā*, and the *Jīvānandanam* (*The Joy of Life*). I discuss other medical and non-medical Sanskrit texts as well, but the lengthiest medical narratives I translate and examine come from these four texts. The *Carakasaṃhitā* is important to each chapter of the book, with the exception of Chapter 6. In the remainder of this chapter I offer descriptions of *Carakasaṃhitā* and the *Suśrutasaṃhitā* and salient information about their histories. I provide an extensive historical discussion of the *Kāśyapasaṃhitā* in Chapter 4, and I treat *The Joy of Life* at length in Chapter 6.

Sources of Āyurveda: *Carakasaṃhitā* and *Suśrutasaṃhitā*

Āyurveda began to take shape around the fourth to fifth centuries B.C.E. Its theories and practices began to be systematized and recorded as treatises from that period forward.[59] The classical ayurvedic sources available to us today are not verbatim reproductions of the works ascribed to the legendary authors Caraka, Suśruta, Bhela, Kaśyapa, Vāgbhaṭa, and others. In fact, these sources were not composed by individual authors or at fixed dates in time; rather, as Tsutomu Yamashita has observed, they were produced "like encyclopedias of which compilation took several centuries."[60] Of the classical Sanskrit manuscripts that survive today, most of them are products of several revisions; others are only partially intact; and none of them, save perhaps the *Carakasaṃhitā*, were likely produced prior to the fourth century C.E., around the time of the Gupta Empire. Steven Engler has suggested that "the [Sanskrit medical] texts were written (at least initially) during the period of political fragmentation, increasing trade, and cultural enrichment between the fall of the Maurya and the rise of the Gupta Empires."[61] Part of Engler's claim is in all likelihood mistaken, for the Mauryan Empire ended around 185 B.C.E., and we have no hard evidence of written medical documents from a period before the Gupta Era (ca. fourth century C.E.—on this end Engler is on the mark), much less anything from before the Common Era. There is evidence of ayurvedic thought, such as the physiologic notion of doṣa (Pali *dosa*), in the Buddhist Pali Canon (*Tripiṭaka*), the earliest portions of which possibly date to the time shortly after the Buddha's death when his disciples began codifying his teachings, circa the mid-fifth century B.C.E.[62] The ayurvedic *saṃhitā*s, however—that is, the collections of medical information in independent written volumes—were not codified until centuries later.

On the whole, the literature of Āyurveda presents a fairly diverse medical tradition. Works claiming to be "ayurvedic" extend for more than two millennia and address subjects ranging from demonology to rhinoplasty to gynecology, among many other medical topics. Although some of the basic principles underlining the sources clearly have common origins, it is nevertheless clear that the processes of development, the central foci, and even the medical "schools" (used in the loosest possible sense) to which each work belongs were different. Regardless, Dominik Wujastyk has argued and persuasively shown that there are a sufficient number of principles and practices that consistently interweave the ayurvedic corpus to warrant reasonably talking about a single, classical Indian tradition of medicine.[63] That tradition of course is Āyurveda, and it crystallized as an organized system of ideas and instructions for medical practitioners and their patients in the early centuries of the Common Era with the redaction of the *Carakasaṃhitā*, which was and continues to be recognized as the tradition's most comprehensively sustained treatise.[64]

There are some historical connections between classical ayurvedic literature and earlier Vedic literature. For example, one finds indications of restorative therapies in Śaunaka's fourth century B.C.E. treatise, the *Ṛgvidhāna* (*Application of the Verses*), which discusses the so-called magical overtones in the canonical *Ṛgveda* (ca. 1550–1200 B.C.E.). A more frequently perceived "medical" connection between the literatures of classical Āyurveda and the Vedas is recognized in the Atharvavedic *Kauśika Sūtra*, which contains numerous passages on healing with mantras and ritual activity. Whereas much of the materia medica in the *Atharvaveda* appears to have evolved into, or served as a kind of botanical baseline for, the materia medica of classical Āyurveda, Kenneth Zysk has shown that very little of the theoretical understanding of health and the empirical approach to disease in the classical tradition can be found in Vedic medicine.[65] In general, the import of the *Atharvaveda* among the classical medical sources is nominal. In the *Suśrutasaṃhitā*, Āyurveda is said to be a supplementary component of the *Atharvaveda*, and the authors of the *Carakasaṃhitā* instruct their students to invoke the *Atharvaveda* as the source of inspiration for their work, should they ever be asked by enquiring physicians.[66] Nevertheless, the physicians' claims of ancestral stock from the *Atharvaveda* do not appear to extend to the clinical practice or anatomical theorizing of classical Āyurveda.[67]

Dating the classical Sanskrit medical sources is an especially thorny and imprecise task. For the reason that there simply is not enough evidence to assign anything more precise than tentative dates for the two works, in the present study I follow Dominik Wujastyk's proposal to situate the sources ascribed to Caraka and Suśruta in relation to one another rather than to try to ascribe precise dates to each: hence, the *Carakasaṃhitā* came first, after which came the *Suśrutasaṃhitā*.[68] Both of these works, it bears repeating, were compiled over long periods of time and revised by many different people. With all of this in mind, I identify the version of the *Carakasaṃhitā* that is available to us today to be a product of the first to second centuries C.E. and the current edition of the *Suśrutasaṃhitā* to be a product of roughly one to two centuries later, so the third to fourth centuries C.E. Along with another compendium, Vāgbhaṭa's

Aṣṭāṅgahṛdayasaṃhitā (ca. the sixth to seventh centuries C.E.), the sources accredited to Caraka and Suśruta are often referred to as the "great trio" (*bṛhattrayī*). That said, I hasten to note that there is no evidence of the use of the term *bṛhattrayī* in the classical sources themselves. The term was coined only recently, perhaps as recently as the nineteenth century, in all likelihood in an effort to organize a kind of ayurvedic canon, with these three texts at the head, followed by another trio, the so-called *laghutrayī*, or "little trio": the *Mādhavanidāna*, *Śārṅgadharasaṃhitā*, and *Bhāvaprakāśa*. To date, the invention and regular use among historians and practitioners of Āyurveda of the classifications of great (*bṛhat-*) and little (*laghu-*) trios in Āyurveda have been neither adequately studied nor connected to an historical event or standard of textual practice in the medical literature itself. Indeed, there is also confusion about whether the third text in the so-called great trio is the *Aṣṭāṅgahṛdayasaṃhitā* or the *Aṣṭāṅgasaṃgrahasaṃhitā*. There is little dispute among scholars that the *Aṣṭāṅgahṛdaya* has been used more widely than the *Aṣṭāṅgasaṃgraha* over the course of Indian history; the far greater number of manuscripts of the *Aṣṭāṅgahṛdaya* than the *Aṣṭāṅgasaṃgraha* in archives and libraries suggests that the *Aṣṭāṅgahṛdaya* has enjoyed a wider circulation throughout the subcontinent than the *Aṣṭāṅgasaṃgraha* has. Yet, interestingly, and no doubt adding to the confusion over the matter, the Indian government has made the *Aṣṭāṅgasaṃgraha* the text of choice on the syllabi of Government Ayurvedic Colleges throughout India.[69]

The *Carakasaṃhitā*: To get an idea of medicine in India before the *Carakasaṃhitā*, the effective cornerstone of classical Indian medicine, Dominik Wujastyk has observed that "we are reduced to searching through books on other—mainly religious—subjects, looking for oblique references which may tell us something about the position of medicine at the time."[70] The *Carakasaṃhitā* is the first fully sustained medical work in Sanskrit literature. It covers a remarkably wide range of material that tends to address theoretical and philosophical questions more than the other classical compendia do.[71] Because of this, and also because the commentarial literature on this work is ample, I rely on the *Carakasaṃhitā* more than the other sources to address various notions in Āyurveda that have a predominantly philosophical or religious history, such as karma, dharma, and the relationship between physical body and transmigratory ātman.

The *Carakasaṃhitā* includes 120 chapters that are spread out over eight sections, each of which varies stylistically in mixtures of verse and prose.[72] The primary focus of the *Carakasaṃhitā* is internal medicine. One of the text's earliest commentators is the seventh-century

C.E. author Jejjaṭa (also spelled Jajjaṭa). His commentary, the *Nirantarapadavyākhyā*, of which only parts have survived, is notable for its rigorous attempt to determine which readings in the text were authentic and which were intercalations.[73] Cakrapāṇidatta (eleventh century C.E.) is the commentator of the *Carakasaṃhitā* most often cited by tradition, and his work, the *Āyurvedadīpikā*, is completely available to us today and highly useful for understanding the root text.[74]

Dominik Wujastyk's careful study of the textual history of the *Carakasaṃhitā* has turned up references to an Indian physician named Caraka in a Chinese text of Buddhist history and legend from the fifth century C.E, the *Saṃyuktaratnapiṭaka Sūtra*.[75] In this text, a medical person named Caraka (along with the Indian poet-philosopher and author of the *Buddhacarita*, Aśvaghoṣa, and a minister, Māṭhara) is a regular companion to a king, Devaputra Kaniṣka. The text of the *Saṃyuktaratnapiṭaka Sūtra* that we have today, however, is a Chinese translation of an original Sanskrit text, which we do not have. Thus, assigning a date to the South Asian original is problematic. Because King Kaniṣka lived during the Kushan Empire in South Asia (first to third centuries C.E.), we can reasonably situate the figure of Caraka to this period. Moreover, we may place the likely origin of the work ascribed to Caraka in the general region of northwestern South Asia, in an area that today includes Kashmir, Afghanistan, Pakistan, and Punjab, given that this general area comprised much of the kingdom of the Kushan Empire.[76] When the *Carakasaṃhitā* was undergoing its early compilation, this area of South Asia was fast becoming a cosmopolitan center of activity and cross-cultural exchanges because of the extensive sections of the Silk Road trading routes that stretched across it. Some of the important centers of knowledge production in this region, of present day Pakistan and Afghanistan such as Taxila and Gandhara, were cynosures for international travelers, merchants, and religious pilgrims coming from as far west as the Mediterranean Sea, the Iranian plateau in Central Asia, the Indian subcontinent, and Japan and China in East Asia. The cosmopolitan activity of the area in which this text was produced and compiled is reflected in the references to people from outside South Asia, including Persians, Chinese, Greeks, and Scythians.[77] The centuries leading up to and after the turn of the Common Era witnessed an expansion of Indian-Buddhist literary culture, which as Sheldon Pollock has suggested, was largely Sanskritic.[78] The Sanskrit medical data of the *Carakasaṃhitā* have long been closely associated with the Buddhist monasteries and medical education centers of Taxila during the Kushan dynasty.[79] Indeed, the legendary physician and teacher of Caraka, Ātreya, was said to have been a teacher there. As a center of pilgrimage for seekers of medical information and training, Taxila in the Kushan Empire was effectively "a link between India and China, and Buddhist missionary activities made the connections even closer," Romila Thapar has written. Indian traders and purveyors of (in this case medical) knowledge, she continues, "were quick to see the advantage of being middlemen in a luxury trade between the Chinese and the centres of the eastern Mediterranean and Byzantium."[80] Caraka's medical compendium was produced in a remarkably diverse cultural area and time. In saying this, we should not overlook the medical sophistication and theoretical insight of Caraka's treatise in its own right, and also note the assured impact of the medical knowledge of the *Carakasaṃhitā* on the Sanskritic literary culture of the period.

Moving beyond the title and into the text, it quickly becomes clear that the name in the title, Caraka, does not refer to an author, but rather to an editor of an earlier text called the *Agniveśa Tantra*. What is more, Caraka was certainly not the last editor of the edition of the *Carakasaṃhitā* that we have today. A person named Dṛḍhabala (ca. fifth century C.E.) subsequently edited Caraka's edition. Dṛḍhabala claims to have added to the *Carakasaṃhita* seventeen chapters on so-called medical substances, which in all likelihood refer to the last seventeen chapters of the Cikitsāsthāna, as well as two entire books, the Kalpa and Siddhi sthānas.[81] We learn from Dṛḍhabala that someone named Caraka expanded and revised an older source composed by one of Ātreya's pupils, Agniveśa, the aforementioned *Agniveśa Tantra*. But who Caraka actually was and how and for what reasons the *Agniveśa Tantra* came to be called the *Carakasaṃhitā* continue to be regular points of debate and speculation.[82]

The style of the *Carakasaṃhitā* is largely didactic, like a medical textbook, though the exhaustiveness of its content is nothing short of encyclopedic. The text is arranged in the form of numerous tutorials of the medical sage, Ātreya Punarvasu, given to Agniveśa. According to tradition, the *Carakasaṃhitā* belongs to the "Ātreya School," which is to say it is part of an elaborate mythological genealogy. The god Brahmā, who first possessed the knowledge for long life that would become the classical medical tradition of Āyurveda, did not create this knowledge, which as Philipp Maas has shown, tradition says "came to the mind of the all-knowing Brahmā all by itself." For example, Cakrapāṇidatta explains that even for Brahmā, "who is the highest teacher [and] who knows all knowledge . . . comprehension of Āyurveda is obtained completely by itself; thus [his knowledge] does not depend upon another teacher."[83] Brahmā then taught Āyurveda to Dakṣa-Prajāpati; Dakṣa-Prajāpati taught it to the divine physicians, the Aśvins, who in turn taught it to the god Indra; Indra is said to have shared the medical knowledge with the sage Bharadvāja, who taught Ātreya Punarvasu; Ātreya Punarvasu then founded a "school," taking on six pupils, Agniveśa, Bhela, Jatūkarṇa, Parāśara, Hārīta, and Kṣārapāṇi, as his first students (as shown in Figure 2).[84]

The *Suśrutasaṃhitā*: The medical treatise ascribed to Suśruta, the *Suśrutasaṃhitā*, is important for many reasons, but above all it is known for its account of surgery.[85] There are over 100 different medical instruments described in this compendium, including scalpels, blunt implements, and forceps. The work contains detailed procedures for the application of caustics, cauterization, and bloodletting using a cow's horn, gourds, and leeches. Most famously, the sixteenth chapter the *Suśrutasaṃhitā* contains extensive discussions on piercing and surgical repair of ears and earlobes and the surgical reconstruction of the nose (i.e., rhinoplasty). For all of its technological innovation in the field of surgery, the procedures expounded in Suśruta's compendium in all likelihood did not continue beyond the middle of the first millennium C.E., and for all intents and purposes surgery has not been part of the ayurvedic tradition ever since.

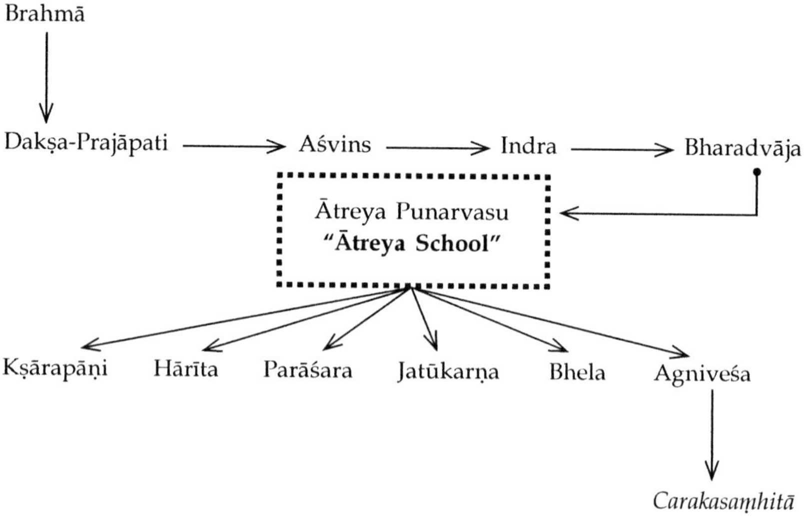

Figure 2. Genealogy of the *Carakasaṃhitā*

The historical person, Suśruta, was purportedly the son of the sage Viśvāmitra and a student of King Divodāsa of Kāśī (later known as Benares, and today called Vārāṇasī). Following Meulenbeld's warning to any prospective chroniclers of the historical Suśruta, it is wise to note that there are many people with the name Suśruta in Sanskrit medical and nonmedical literature who may or may not be the same person as the namesake of this Sanskrit medical work.[86] In nonmedical literature, for instance, a surgeon named Suśruta in the Anuśāsana Parvan of the *Mahābhārata* has the same familial profile as the Suśruta of Āyurveda.[87] The *Garuḍa Purāṇa* mentions a Suśruta who was a son of Viśvāmitra, and the *Agni Purāṇa* states that a man by the name of Suśruta was a student of King Divodāsa and that he studied the arts of human and equine medicine.[88] Occasionally, when numerous Sanskrit sources are taken into account to determine familial relations of quasi-historical figures, from one historical period to another, relationships and personal profiles appear to change. Such is the case with Suśruta's relationship to Viśvāmitra. K. R. Srikanta Murthy has pointed out that the *Ṛgveda* and the *Rāmāyaṇa* both say that Viśvāmitra is the father of Suśruta, yet it is fairly well accepted that the Viśvāmitras of these two works are not one and the same figure.[89]

According to the *Suśrutasaṃhita* itself, a physician named Suśruta acquired his medical knowledge as a student in the "Dhanvantari School," which, along with the Ātreya School, is one of the two dominant medical traditions in classical Āyurveda. The mythological lineage of the Dhanvantari School is identical to the Ātreya School up to the god Indra, at which point, instead of the knowledge of Āyurveda being imparted to Bharadvāja, Indra is said to have taught it to Dhanvantari, whom, Meulenbeld explains, tradition recognizes as Divodāsa, king of Kāśī.[90] In the city of Kāśī on the banks of the Ganges River, Divodāsa (also known as Dhanvantari and Kāśīrāja) then established his own "school" of medicine by teaching seven pupils: Aupadhenava, Vaitaraṇa, Aurabhra, Pauṣkalāvata, Karavīrya, Gopurarakṣita, and Suśruta (as shown in Figure 3).[91]

In its present form, the *Suśrutasaṃhitā* has 120 chapters divided across five broad sections; a supplementary appendix, the Uttaratantra, consisting of 66 chapters, brings the total number of chapters in the work to 186. For decades scholars have agreed that the Uttaratantra is a late addition to the original five sections of the *Suśrutasaṃhitā* and that one of the text's redactors likely added it. But who that person was remains uncertain.[92] Among the commentators on the *Suśrutasaṃhitā*, Jejjaṭa was among the first. Jejjaṭa's commentary has been only partially preserved, and the name of his work is not known.[93]

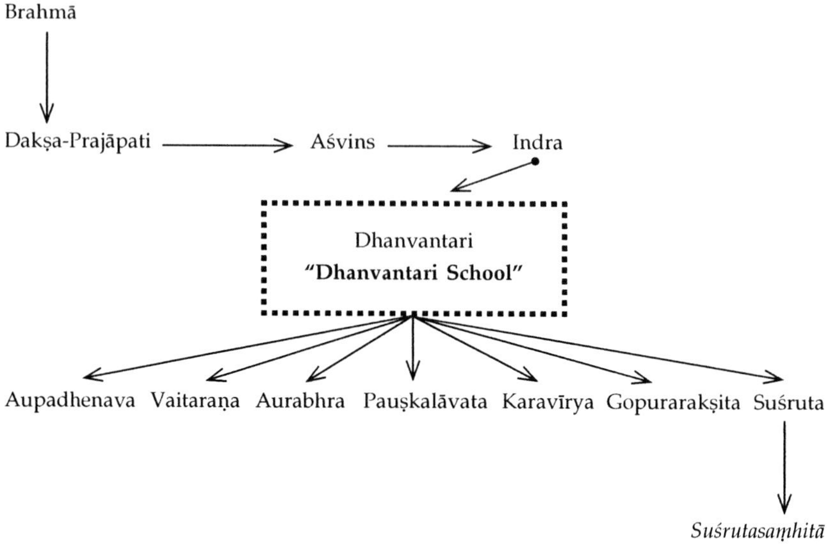

Figure 3. Genealogy of the *Suśrutasaṃhitā*

Apart from Jejjaṭa, commentaries on *Suśruta* include Cakrapāṇidatta's *Bhānumatī* (eleventh century C.E.), which we do not have today, and the extant and widely cited *Nibandhasaṃgraha* of Ḍalhaṇa (twelfth century C.E.).[94] In the *Nibandhasaṃgraha*, Ḍalhaṇa explains that a person named Nāgārjuna redacted the *Suśrutasaṃhitā*, although he provides precious little information about whether this Nāgārjuna was the famous Buddhist Madhyamaka philosopher (ca. 150–250 C.E.) of the same name or a different Nāgārjuna, such as the famous military surgeon during the Gupta Era or one of the many other Nāgārjunas in South Asia in the early centuries of the Common Era.[95]

Is There an Ayurvedic Way of Thinking (about the Body)?

In 1979 Francis Zimmermann significantly problematized the ways in which historians of Indian medicine understand the body in Āyurveda and discuss somatic descriptions in the Sanskrit medical sources. Taking a comparative look at the history of medicine in the West, in "Remarks on the Conception of the Body in Ayurvedic Medicine," he declared that "there is no real anatomy" in Āyurveda. What Zimmermann meant by this assertion speaks to a particular way of thinking in Āyurveda and the Sanskrit sources of the tradition that, to riff on A. K. Ramanujan's famous inquiry, connotes a distinctly ayurvedic way of thinking about the human body that is at once "context-sensitive" and "context-free."[96] On the one hand, Zimmermann's eloquent and innovative research on Āyurveda in his short 1979 article and numerous publications thereafter forced scholars of Indian medicine, like no one had before him, to interpret the ways in which the Sanskrit sources depict the human body as a highly structured and contextualized site. The body is a frame for the fundamental confluence and interchange of vital fluids and internal somatic mechanisms, Zimmermann showed, which are impacted by various and sundry things like the seasons, geography, and diet (each of which has its own properties and contexts); these influential contexts in turn produce enormous sensitivity to context in the medical work of diagnosis, prescription, and the preparation of medicine. Yet on the other hand, Zimmermann's investigation into the epistemology of Āyurveda also suggested that ayurvedic literature tends toward context-free thinking about the body: despite an intricate relationship and reciprocal dependency with its society and ecology through such conduits as humoral makeup, seasonal cycles, family and environment, the body is also unencumbered and fluid in ways that contrast to anatomical thinking in biomedicine. Where Ramanujan saw context-free thinking in Indian culture, for Zimmerman there is in Āyurveda indeterminacy:

> I wish to determine the epistemological position of anatomical knowledge. In a word, there is no real anatomy; the humours are vital fluids, and the frame of the body is a network of channels through which vital fluids must be kept flowing in the right direction. The nature and function of organs like the heart, which is the centre of this network, stay indeterminate.[97]

There might not be real anatomy in Āyurveda. But there is physiology. And there is pathology. There is rationative concern with the functioning of the body and a careful investigation of what are considered to be somatic normality and abnormality. These two types of medical study are based on processes and currents. Following Zimmermann's lead, I would suggest they move ayurvedic thinking (or epistemology, as Zimmermann originally framed it) in the direction of contextually free thinking alongside, or perhaps as the result of, the contextually sensitive nature of medical knowledge that organizes thinking about the appropriateness of things like season and geography in the designation of health.[98]

The nature of chart talk in ayurvedic literature—that is, the propensity for aphoristic explanations, botanical litanies, and pinpointable descriptions with fixed objectives—generates a literary *mise en scène* in the Sanskrit classics that obfuscates the complicated epistemology Zimmermann identified. Indeed, Zimmermann's trenchant hermeneutical method taught us that when one reads across the medical literature, seeing a comprehensive tradition comprised of texts that are in conversation with one another, and when one has sufficient knowledge of the commonly unstated theories supporting the tradition's chart talk, the body in ayurvedic literature emerges as an entity that is neither ever static nor independent. It constantly reforms itself according to the various streams of context to which it is subjected. The ways in which the classical Indian medical authors thought about the body moved through an ideational process that syncs nicely with Ramanujan's description of Indian knowing, which he described as "a continuity, a constant flow (the etymology of *saṁsāra*!) of substance from context to object, from non-self to self."[99] It is a flow between body and context—season, diet, land, society, religion—that signals a physiology larger than an individual's bodily functioning, a physiology brilliantly allegorized in Ānandarāya's *The Joy of Life*, which I discuss in Chapter 6, and analogized in cosmic terms in the illness narrative of the king's disease, which I examine in Chapter 5. Undergirding ayurvedic thinking about how a body works and whether it works well or sputters due to illness is the idea that a person's physiologic health is contingent on its position and relationship of exchange with this larger context of soil, air, altitude, vegetation, other people, cultural institutions (religion, politics, medicine, economy), animals, and so on. The numerous contexts recounted in the Sanskrit medical sources that determine important somatic states, such as health and sickness, operate in a field of syntactic meaning that "yields finally a *sphoṭa*, an explosion, a meaning which is beyond sequence and time," in the classic sense that Ramanujan saw thinking function in "traditional" cultures like India.[100] Ayurvedic thinking about the body at once insists on the need for a sequence of rules and parameters and denies the stricture of context-sensitive structures. The basic building blocks of the body—doṣas, basic substances (*dhātus*), and elemental *rasas*, "tastes"—are found across the animal, vegetable, and mineral kingdoms, as well as throughout the cosmos. The compilers of ayurvedic literature wove together a somatic sensibility that is "neither the unique, nor the universal," as Ramanujan put it, but one knowledge system with two types of emphases.[101]

Zimmermann's arguments about the conception of the body in Āyurveda are significant, and at the time he made them they were highly innovative within the study of Indian medical history. They are also useful to bear in mind, and to ponder briefly, in the present study. In saying there is no "real anatomy" in Āyurveda, Zimmermann refers specifically to the biomedical view that anatomy is a science of representing the shape and structure of an organism and its parts. Zimmermann was absolutely correct to note that we do not have illustrations of the body in the classical medical literature (although there may have been images in the classical period, they simply did not survive transmission through the centuries). Zimmermann explained the task of the ayurvedic authors to put their thinking about the body into language thusly:

> To describe the parts of the body and their functions, the Sanskrit texts make use of the most unmarked words: to go, to stay, to nourish, to support. . . . There is no map nor topography of the body but only an *economy*, that is to say, fluids going in or coming out, residing in some *āśraya*, "recipient" (organs are conceived of as recipients), or flowing through some *srotas*, "channel."[102]

We have to rely on verbal representations to understand how the compilers of the medical tradition understood the composition of the body, some of which I recounted earlier in this chapter. In modern biomedicine, the science of anatomy involves dissection, the methodical cutting up of a body for the purpose of displaying its internal structure. The standard type of presentation of the body found in modern medical textbooks like *Gray's Anatomy*, for instance, is the product of generations of accrued knowledge based on anatomical dissection. Dissection is very much a part of "real anatomy" in modern biomedical discourse. Could the lack of dissection in ayurvedic literature lead one to suggest that there is no real anatomy in Āyurveda? Or is it anachronistic to speak of dissection in Indian history and the Sanskrit sources of Āyurveda? Modern biomedical dissection per se is not common in the Sanskrit medical sources. Nevertheless surgical techniques and somatic knowledge in the *Suśrutasaṃhitā* indicate that among at least a circle of premodern Indian physicians, somatic investigation involved elements of dissection and analysis common in biomedical anatomy. Considerably earlier than the compendium of Suśruta, dissective passages relating to ritual animal sacrifices occur in the *Ṛgveda*. Most notably, in three verses of *Ṛgveda*, Book 1, there is a famous account of how to carve up the sacrificial horse of the ancient *aśvamedha*, "horse sacrifice," which could serve as a step-by-step guide for the ritual dissector.[103] To be sure, Indologists like A. F. Rudolf Hoernle, Kenneth Zysk, Heinrich Zimmer and, to a lesser extent, A. L. Basham has each documented what he refers to as anatomy in Indian literature and history.[104] One should not be content with a scholar's designation of "anatomy" in the ancient Indian world as sufficient evidence for the existence of a bona fide anatomical science, of course. Zimmermann's provocative suggestion is indication of that.

I do not dispute Zimmermann's claim that the Sanskrit medical sources emphasize a somatic "economy," in the sense that classical ayurvedic bodytalk often amounts to an ordering of physiologic processes and pathological concepts, rather than a systematically displayed assembly of calibrated parts that contribute to (or detract from) a bodily unit. In an effort to understand fully the history of thought on the body in Āyurveda, it is worth reiterating that Zimmermann's primary concern was "to determine an ayurvedic epistemological position of anatomical knowledge."[105] As I explain momentarily, the underlying value and brilliance of the assertion that Āyurveda has "no real anatomy," for all of the important philological wrangling that could result from a study of such a position, is more methodological than semantic. That said, there is another angle to the anatomy question in Āyurveda that I would like to add before getting to the debt we owe Zimmermann for his work on the body in Indian medical history.

Before declaring the lack of real anatomy in Āyurveda, Zimmermann argued that the dominant conception of the body in classical ayurvedic medicine is based on the concepts of the three doṣas and six rasas. These concepts dominate ayurvedic theories of the body, in Zimmermann's view, because they remain unchanging throughout the literature.[106] The significance of doṣa and rasa in Indian medicine can hardly be overstated. Yet there is a view of somatic structure in Āyurveda that dominates the tradition's contemporary practice among Malayali physicians in the southwest Indian state of Kerala, which complicates Zimmermann's early ideas about an ayurvedic epistemology of the body and suggests a particular modern ayurvedic way of thinking about the body. It is based on theory in the *Carakasaṃhitā*, in particular the concepts of quality (*guṇa*) and action (*karman*) rather than doṣa and rasa.[107] In my experience working with ayurvedic physicians in central Kerala who treat their patients according to this system, they regard it as ayurvedic anatomy. This conceptual framework structures how these Indian physicians think about the body. Take the Sanskrit word for "bone," *asthi*. The translation of *asthi* into English "bone" is problematic according to the "quality-action theory" because "bone" does not sufficiently express the breadth of the meaning of the Sanskrit word *asthi*.[108] The main quality of *asthi* is firmness and sturdiness, and its predominant action (*karman*) is support. A physician determines a substance that has the primary quality of firmness and the primary activity of support to be *asthi*. This substance may or may not be bone, but it positively refers to a body part that in some way provides support and firmness to the body, which of course bones can and often do. But cartilage, too, has the same defining quality and action. In general, *asthi* in ayurvedic thinking contributes more to somatic design and bodily functioning than bone does in biomedical anatomy. There is arguably more flexibility in ayurvedic thinking about the body than there is in biomedical anatomy. But in the *Carakasaṃhitā*'s important system of identification and classification of bodily substances according to quality and action, there appears to be a very real kind of anatomy in Āyurveda.

In seeing no real anatomy in classical Āyurveda, perhaps Zimmermann set his sights too narrowly on fluidity—which he took to be the Indian counterpart of biomedical physiology and pathology—rather than any probable sense of fixity in the ayurvedic body—which he presumably took to be the equivalent of biomedical anatomy. What is at issue here is perhaps not anatomy as such, but the very duality of epistemic focus on both bodily physiology and cosmic physiology in the sense that Ramanujan identified two coterminous currents of thought in Indian cultural history. Looking across Zimmermann's oeuvre, it is clear that he, more than any scholar of Indian medical history and literature, has illustrated the profound breadth and depth of ayurvedic thinking about the body as but one fluid part of a universal stream of being. This is part of ayurvedic thinking about the body, to be sure. But if we move our analysis of the body in Āyurveda too quickly away from the specifics of internal somatic associations and organization—away from where Ramanujan said "context-sensitivity rules and binds"—to the medical tradition's homologues between body and cosmos, cosmological physiologies, so to speak—where "the dream is to be free of context"[109]—the correspondences between the constituents of body and worldly material can negate the very notion of an internal and consistent ayurvedic anatomy. The correspondences are of course there in the medical literature, and they speak to the potential effects of people's environments on their diet and routines, maintenance of bodily integrity, and abilities to sustain and achieve health. That ayurvedic medicine claims the same elements of the cosmos also make up the body does not of necessity mean that Āyurveda lacks focus on somatic substance or anatomy. The literature asserts a definite set of inter-reliant parts that comprise the structure of the human body. If we must translate using biomedical terms, in English, I would suggest that that the body in classical ayurvedic literature may be reasonably called anatomical.

Zimmermann's statement about ayurvedic thinking on the body gives rise to some very important methodological issues in the textual and historical study of Indian medicine. On the one hand, his position calls into question the suitability of non-Indian languages, especially totalizing biomedical categories such as anatomy, for translating the literature and practices of Āyurveda. Translation is never foolproof. *Traduttore traditore*, as the Italians say, "the translator [is a] traitor." Or perhaps more suitable here is the Hungarian adage *fordítás ferdítés*, "translation [is] distortion." It would of course be best if an author could always be involved in her or his translations. But that is rarely possible. When translation involves great gaps in time and place, as well as complex elements of knowledge systems like anatomy, the task of translation becomes exceedingly difficult. Are we translating irresponsibly when we use the term "anatomy" to explicate ayurvedic thinking about the body? In using the term, are we (those of us steeped in a biomedical culture) reading into this classical Sanskritic medical tradition a type of scientific thought that we presume ought to be there because it is so basic to modern establishment biomedicine around the globe? Zimmermann's careful scholarship on Āyurveda challenges us to consider these questions whenever we attempt to translate the textual sources of the tradition. There will be scholars who adamantly oppose translating Āyurveda's Sanskrit technical terms, insisting instead on retaining the original terms in Sanskrit and/or offering lengthy descriptions of these terms to address their many contextual particularities. There also will be scholars who translate these terms into modern languages. Some will do so willingly because of the intellectual and cultural benefits that bringing previously unknown knowledge of "other peoples" to a wide audience can occasion; some will do so begrudgingly because of the inherent imprecision and potential misinterpretations involved. Although Zimmermann was not exactly decrying the practice of translation in his 1979 article, his probe of the anatomical epistemology of Āyurveda throws light on, and serves to upset our predispositions about, the imprecision inherent in translation and the biases that we, in the modern Western world, might bring to our translations and interpretations of the classical Indian world.

Even more instructive than his problematization of medical anatomy and its epistemological bases is Zimmermann's use of "real" to qualify anatomy: "In a word, there is no real anatomy." Could he have thought a systematic study of the human body and its parts, with or without active dissection, in the classical Indian world did not actually exist as a mode of inquiry? That is not likely. Anyone familiar with his work on the body and knowledge structures in Āyurveda would readily know that even he sees a kind of, or something like, anatomical structure and organization in the literature of Āyurveda. Perhaps that is the lesson to be taken from his use of "real." The word implies authorial perspective and a situatedness that is steeped in language that purports to relate what is true. Āyurveda might have an anatomy, but it is not anatomy in a modern biomedical sense. Herein lies the groundbreaking quality of Zimmermann's 1979 article. Ever so subtly yet compellingly, his keen observations of the ways in which the medical compilers of Āyurveda envisioned the cynosure of their medical system, the human body, pushed historians of Indian medicine to consider whether or not biomedical terms may be gainfully used (or whether they should be used at all) to explicate Indian medical concepts, paradigms, and processes.

If Zimmermann is correct and there is no anatomy in classical Āyurveda, then scholars of Indian medicine need to rethink the long-standing use of biomedical categories in the study of Indian medicine. Instead of using biomedical models and analytical categories to explain Indian medical practice and literature, Zimmermann's claim indirectly challenges us to search for and understand the tradition's own method for explaining the human body, in theory and in practice, as a "closed" and autonomous physiologic unit as well as a system of health and disease "open" to the influences of its environment. How do the Sanskrit medical texts account for the fact that, as the body turns so turns the medical knowledge of Āyurveda? How did classical Indian vaidyas, who dealt principally with the maintenance of health and deterrence of disease, come to know and conceive of their subject, the patient, whose ailing body is the lodestone for their inquiries into health and sickness? One of the ways the medical authors dealt with the uniquely ayurvedic way of thinking about the body as both an open and closed unit, a complex physiologic system that is constantly in flux as its contexts change, was to narrativize the body and the life of the patient. The narrative side of the classical Sanskrit medical literature has received little to no attention in scholarship on Indian medical history. As I show in the following chapters, illness narratives in Āyurveda not only illustrate in a lucid manner the ways in which the body has been distinctively conceived in Indian medical circles, but they also scrupulously interweave Indian medical thinking about the body with Indian religion and social construction.

Chapter 3

Fever

Few diseases in Sanskrit medical literature are more forbidding than fever (*jvara*). In Chapter 2 I explained that in the literature of classical Āyurveda, diseases typically assail just the body, just the mind, or just the sense organs. The *Carakasaṃhitā* advances this general principle with few exceptions. Fever, for its frequency and doggedness, stands as the foremost exception. It is a titan among the legion of diseases examined in the compendium of Caraka, for it afflicts all three: the body, the mind, and the sense organs.[1] It is an indefatigable and lifelong enemy to every human being. In fact, fever literally frames human existence according to the *Carakasaṃhitā*, for it bathes every person in a kind of amnesia-inducing darkness at the beginning and the end of life.[2] What is more, although fever causes physical and mental suffering among humanity, the *Carakasaṃhitā* bluntly explains that no living being is immune to fever's advance: "The distinguishing mark of fever is pain of the body and mind. And fever's reach torments every living creature."[3]

In English, the word "fever" can denote a few different things. An excessively elevated bodily temperature is perhaps the most common meaning of the word. By extension from this meaning, fever was once a moniker for blacksmiths, forgers, and other such professionals whose work involved sustained close contact with hot iron and other metals. In biomedical professions specifically, fever is a generic term denoting a group of diseases that share the common symptoms of elevated temperature and similar tissue deterioration, and each specific type of disease also carries a distinguishing label, such as yellow fever, scarlet fever, typhoid fever, and so forth. Furthermore, in English, fever can indicate a state of vigorous, nervous excitement or agitation, suggesting that fever in some way pertains to a person's behavior or modal states of being in the world. In grammatical terms, fever is as much verbal as it is nominal, so that to be saddled with fever is in a sense to burn. This dynamism captures the general meaning of *jvara* the medical authors deploy in the Sanskrit narratives of fever. The principal idea expressed in these stories is that people get *jvara* because of reprehensible social comportment and activities that ensue from poor self-understanding and bad decisions. In the *Carakasaṃhitā*'s narrative of fever, the lengthiest of the classical medical narratives of fever, the primary causes of fever in the world are social and religious behaviors. Yet beyond that, simply by virtue of being human, irrespective of one's behavior, the text declares that every person experiences fever at least twice in one's lifetime: at birth and at death.

The authors of the *Carakasaṃhitā* assign a gravity and ubiquity to fever in various places throughout the compendium's eight sections. In this chapter, I take up specific parts of their discussion, focusing on an extended narrative about the origin of fever in the compendium's section on therapeutics (*cikitsāsthāna*).[4] It is a recycled version of a popular Hindu myth, commonly called "The Destruction of Dakṣa's Sacrifice" or simply "Dakṣa's Sacrifice." This medical articulation of the Dakṣa story connects the outbreak of fever with the poor performance of a Hindu ritual, which the text's compilers perceived to oppose proper and commonsensical behavior. The use of this Hindu story appears to have been an attempt to adapt the empiricism of Āyurveda to the religious environment in India in the early centuries of the first millennium C.E., when the *Carakasaṃhitā* as we have it today was redacted. The narrative also appears to have been a vehicle with which to posit a uniquely medical commentary on two important religious concepts in Hinduism: karma and dharma.

Addressing a great deal more than human biology, the narrative of fever in the *Carakasaṃhitā* is an exposition on the ways in which people should act, given their knowledge of religious practice and their physical abilities. The story of "Dakṣa's Sacrifice" calls attention to the power and consequences of people's actions, that is, their karma, in the present lifetime—rather than actions in former lifetimes, which the karma concept also entails—as an important basis for explaining health and illness. Using narrative logic as the means to press this point, the story makes the case that the relationship between the maintenance of one's socioreligious duties, or one's dharma, and one's resistance or susceptibility to disease is reciprocally causal: a person's biophysical circumstances are contingent on the quality of his or her ethics and religious practice; conversely, a person's ethics and religious practice are only as effective as the quality of his or her physical health. The underlying message is that when people act in the world, they create forces on others and objects around them, sometimes unintentionally and sometimes on purpose; the objects and people who are affected by the force of a person's actions subsequently exert a counterforce of equal measure, but in the opposite direction. This cycle of cause and effect both stems from the individual and returns to the individual. Health or a lack of health, so the logic of the story goes, depends on the ethical quality and religious propriety (or dharma) of the actions and behaviors (or karma) that people produce in society.[5]

In the medical context, "Dakṣa's Sacrifice" not only serves the function of connecting religious ethics and somatic well-being by focusing on religious sacrifice (*yajña*) and dharmic fulfillment, but it also homologizes physical well-being with religious sacrifice. Thus, proper treatment of the body necessitates attention and maintenance akin to care and governance given to a well-performed sacrifice. Just as a successful sacrifice requires careful attention to ritual protocol, the achievement of a long life free of disease demands that people ensure that their actions are consistent with their social and religious duties. The upshot of a well-performed sacrifice is that sacrificers get what they desire; the payoff of a long-lived life free from disease is that people may achieve all or a combination of Hinduism's four valid aims of human life: kāma, artha, dharma, and release (*mokṣa*) from the cycle of rebirth and redeath.[6]

"Dakṣa's Sacrifice" has a long history in Sanskrit literature. I look at some of the nonmedical variants of the narrative in this chapter to supply some of the information that is absent in the *Carakasaṃhitā*'s medical version. Although I concentrate primarily on the fever narrative in the text's section on therapeutics, I also investigate variant accounts of the story, or more precisely miniature portraits of the story, in the *Carakasaṃhitā*, *Bhelasaṃhitā*, *Suśrutasaṃhitā*, *Aṣṭāṅgahṛdayasaṃhitā*, and *Mādhavanidāna*.[7]

The Narrative of Fever

In the retelling of "Dakṣa's Sacrifice" in the section on therapeutics of the *Carakasaṃhitā*, there are two main characters: Dakṣa-Prajāpati and Rudra. Both are well-known figures and appear in a variety of stories throughout Hindu mythology. The name Dakṣa-Prajāpati means "Able Lord of Creatures." The Sanskrit word *dakṣa* has multiple meanings: adjectivally, it means "able" and "intelligent"; nominally, it means "ability" and "intelligence." A *prajāpati* is a "lord of creatures." Often, though not always, Dakṣa is depicted as one of the progenitors of the human race, properly known as a *prajāpati*.[8] He frequently belongs to a group of seers, who, depending on the source, spontaneously materialize out of the thoughts of Brahmā, the Creator, just prior to the creation of the cosmos.[9] In the *Ṛgveda*, Dakṣa is one of the Ādityas, or offspring of Aditi, while remarkably, Aditi is also said to be Dakṣa's daughter.[10] As we saw in the preceding chapter, medical legend holds that Brahmā was the first to receive the knowledge system for achieving long life, Āyurveda, and that he taught it directly to Dakṣa-Prajāpti. Dakṣa is also the name of the father of Satī, Ambikā, Umā, Rohiṇī, and other wives of the gods, most notably of the god Śiva.[11] Many characters named Dakṣa in Sanskrit literature display a noticeably sexual disposition, marked by lust for women, and on one occasion, Dakṣa is said to be incestuously attracted to his daughter. On account of this licentious itch, in many stories Dakṣa is decapitated, and his former head replaced with the head of a goat, which is an animal that recurrently symbolizes lust and craving in Sanskrit literature.[12]

The Sanskrit name Rudra means "Fearsome One." The word *rudra* has the adjectival meaning of "terrible, fearsome, or howling" and the nominal meaning of "growler" or "howler." In the *Ṛgveda*, Rudra is a storm deity—or a group of storm deities called the Rudras (also known as the Maruts)—and the god of medicinal herbs.[13] Throughout the Vedic literature Rudra is a baleful and shadowy deity whose temperament swings from the creative to the destructive quite liberally. In the *Atharvaveda* he is explicitly linked with the fever god Takman as well as the human manifestation of fever, *takmán* (I return to this association momentarily).[14] Rudra is also the Vedic deity most frequently identified, perhaps overly so, as the chief mythological antecedent of the god Śiva, the so-called Destroyer in the classical Hindu "trinity" (*trimūrti*—alongside Brahmā the Creator and Viṣṇu the Preserver). The name Śiva is never mentioned in the *Ṛgveda*, although in the *Yajurveda* Śiva is mentioned in connection with Rudra.[15] In the Purāṇas and in the *Mahābhārata*, the Sanskrit poets regularly invoke Śiva by the name Rudra.[16] In the *Carakasaṃhitā*'s narrative account of fever, the names Rudra and Śiva hang together unpredictably, as the story's authors freely interchange the names. Additionally, the narrative contains three other epithets for Rudra-Śiva: Maheśvara ("Great Lord"), Paśupati ("Lord of Creatures"), and Mahātma ("Great Self").

The following is a translation of the *Carakasaṃhitā*'s narrative description of fever in its section on therapeutics. Ātreya Punarvasu narrates the story to his pupil, Agniveśa.[17]

> It has been said the condition of fever arises from attachment. Yet earlier, in the section on primary causes, it was

> also pointed out that fever arises from the intense anger of the god Rudra.
>
> In the Second Cosmic Age, the Tretā Yuga, Rudra made a vow of non-anger for 1,000 divine years [= 360,000 human years]. Taking advantage of the situation, the demons, who derive nourishment from the obstruction of people's religious observances, hastened to block Rudra's vow. Though Dakṣa saw this, he disregarded it. Furthermore, when he was preparing his sacrifice, Dakṣa did not arrange the fixed share of offerings for Maheśvara, even though the gods implored him to do so. And even though the sacrificial oblations offered to Śiva and the hymns of the *Ṛgveda* sung to Paśupati ensure a successful sacrifice, Dakṣa omitted them during his worship.
>
> When Rudra's vow of non-anger ended, he learned of Dakṣa's misconduct, and he became furious. He opened the eye on his forehead, and fire erupted forth scorching the demons [who had irritated him during his vow]. Then, for the purpose of destroying Dakṣa's sacrifice, Rudra created a child, who was ablaze with fire of his anger. This child destroyed the sacrifice, and the excruciating feeling of being in flames seized the throngs of gods and people in all directions.
>
> The gods and seven Vedic sages then sang hymns of praise to the all-pervading deity [Rudra-Śiva] to put him in an auspicious (*śiva*) state-of-mind. Upon learning that all living creatures were in Śiva's esteem, the fierce anger-fire [that was Śiva's child][18]—standing with hands cupped in supplication, bearing a weapon made of ash, with three dreadful heads and nine-eyes, ensconced in garlands of fire, irascible, with dwarfish legs and a dwarfish belly—approached the god and said: "What should I do for you now?"
>
> Rudra replied to his anger: "You will become fever in the world at the start of life, at death, and among people who act improperly."[19]

Juxtaposed with the standard chart talk of the *Carakasaṃhitā*, this narrative is quite remarkable. The passages immediately preceding and following the story of "Dakṣa's Sacrifice" discuss fever according to climate, diet, season, and other perceptibly discernable factors that could verify pathology. Elsewhere in the compendium we learn that fever strikes in eight different ways and with varying degrees of severity. Cakrapāṇidatta says that contributory factors of fever in the *Carakasaṃhitā* are of two types: those pertaining to imminent causes, such as physical constitution or aggravated bodily humors, and those pertaining to more distant causes, such as quality of available food or time of year, which may in the future vitiate the bodily humors.[20] This is all to say that sooner or later fever is linked to the body's humoral distribution in some way.[21] How, then, do we begin to make sense of this narrative explanation for what is characteristically a physical malady? What explanatory function does the Dakṣa story perform in this medical text? Sacrificial foibles of a legendary character from a popular myth at one and the same time appear to reflect and cause fever.[22] The patient in the story, Dakṣa, embodies notions of improper disposition and activity, while the story line indirectly suggests the importance of behavior in the prevention of sickness.

The Structure of Fever in Narrative Discourse

Tailored to the task of explaining the origin of fever, the rendition of "Dakṣa's Sacrifice" in the *Carakasaṃhitā* is a kind of narrative patchwork that consists of isolable units, each of which has an independent history outside this medical text. A look at their non-medical backgrounds, and the ways in which they have been situated in the medical framework, can help to illuminate the literary form the narrative has taken, as well as its apparent function, in this ayurvedic work.

In the first two lines of the narrative, there are two important declarations about fever that could, at first blush, appear unrelated. Fever, the text explains, is a consequence of attachment, *parigraha*, yet its source is the god Rudra's anger. These two statements and their syntactic relationship are critical to understanding the form and function of the narrative of fever in this classical medical work. Let us first look at the short reference about Rudra's anger. This is in effect a miniature version of the Dakṣa narrative, which we can identify within a larger cycle of Dakṣa narratives within the context of the Sanskrit medical literature. The short statement "Fever arises from the intense anger of the god Rudra" may be read, following Wendy Doniger's mythic hermeneutics, as a "minimyth."[23] As its name suggests, a minimyth expresses a great deal of information in only a few words. With great economy, a minimyth expresses an entire story line and setting and conveys an intrinsic meaning that typically is widely known. To expand a minimyth is to create, predictably, what

Doniger calls a "maximyth." The maximyth is fuller, in an ornamental sense, than the minimyth because it relies on idiomatic turns of phrase and creative abstraction to communicate specific meanings subtly and imaginatively. A maximyth explicitly expresses culturally and contextually particular details that the minimyth merely evokes. Details added to the basic storyline often allude to specific cultural categories like geography, local politics, religion and ritual practice, science, aesthetics, and the like, all of which might be known to only certain social groups.[24]

An intertextual reference at the beginning of the Dakṣa story ("Yet earlier in the text, in the section on primary causes . . .") draws our attention (". . . it was also pointed out . . .") to the minimyth (". . . fever arises from the intense anger of the god Rudra"), which the following maximyth expands. The minimyth is skeletal, devoid of detail, and short on words. All the same, it is a fully formed narrative. With the addition of narrative details (for example, the important element that Rudra sires a child out of his third eye to destroy Dakṣa's sacrifice and to become fever in the world), the minimythic kernel effectively pops, bursting forth with new details and meaning as a maximyth. The base meaning remains, but the retelling of the story suggests a vivid and particular context in which to substantiate the base story.

Minimyths of the creation of fever springing from Rudra's anger, or slight variations of it, occur in four Sanskrit medical sources other than the *Carakasaṃhitā*, as well as in another location in the *Carakasaṃhitā* itself. I present them below, with the recurring minimyth highlighted in bold. Each minimyth occurs in the context of a discussion on fever, although not one of the following five sources enlarges the base myth to the extent that the compendium of Caraka does in its section on therapeutics (*cikitsāsthāna*).

Carakasaṃhitā, Nidānasthāna

> **Fever is produced from Maheśvara's anger.** It takes the breath of all breathing beings. It produces heat in the body, sense organs, and mind. It weakens one's intellect, strength, happiness, and determination. It causes fatigue, exhaustion, unconsciousness, and occludes the intake of food. It is called "fever" because it causes bodies to become hot. No other disease is as severe, as great a misfortune, or as dif-

ficult to treat as this. It is the chief of all diseases. It is described with many turns of phrase consistent with the diverse species of animals. All breathing beings are born with fever, and all die with fever. It is an enormous mental stupefaction. Therefore, embodied beings overcome [with fever] do not remember any previous bodily acts. In death, fever takes away the breath of all breathing beings.[25]

Bhelasaṃhitā, Cikitsāsthāna

Some physicians have said intermittent fever is due primarily to the vāta-doṣa. Some say it is caused by a combination effect [of all three doṣas]. Others link it to the pitta-doṣa. Still others say it is born of the kapha-doṣa. Some identify its source as demonic beings. People who have doubts about the [existence of the] gods say it is on account of stellar eclipses at the time of one's birth. Like this, the opinions of the authors of the śāstras are of various types. I, Bhelācārya, will speak about this fever with causes born from a combination effect. . . . [Having outlined the vitiation sequence of the combined doṣic effect of an intermittent fever, Bhela declares:] . . . So it is, **this fever in the body of living beings is the dreadful Maheśvara**. Therefore the clear-sighted physician should make every effort to placate Maheśvara.[26]

Suśrutasaṃhitā, Uttaratantra

Fever is born from the fire of Rudra's anger and torments all living creatures. Among different types of creatures it is known by different names. At the beginning of birth and at death it runs its course through the body. For this reason it is called the king of all diseases. No one apart from gods and men can endure it. Despite being human, by virtue of one's actions, one can become godlike. But that person is shaken from the heavens and reverts back to a human state. Human beings thus endure fever through [their propensity to experience] the state of being divine. All other animals afflicted by fever perish.[27]

Aṣṭāṅgahṛdayasaṃhitā, Nidānasthāna

Now we will explain the primary causes of fever. About this, Ātreya and the great sages said: "Fever is the father of the diseases; it is evil; and it is death. It devours vitality, and it marks the end of life. **It is the anger that sprang from the upper eye of Rudra**, the destroyer of Dakṣa's sacrifice. It is the delusion one experiences at the time of birth and death. It is characterized by unbearable heat, and it arises because of improper behavior. A ferocious thing, fever exists among various species by various names."[28]

Mādhavanidāna, Jvaranidāna

Dakṣa's disrespect **incensed Rudra, whose breath gave birth to fever.**[29]

Taken together, these five accounts offer a unique glimpse into how a specific body of Sanskrit literature—medical compendia—use narrative logic to explain disease. As a group of literary discourses contributing to the same body of "knowledge for long life" that is Āyurveda, these five passages also illustrate the intertextual relationship between the ayurvedic compendia.

Etiologic minimyths of fever in the Sanskrit medical sources—that is, variations of "fever originates out of Rudra's anger"—effectively serve the same purpose as maximyths, that of explaining the source(s) of *jvara*. For historians working with ancient texts, there are some frequently followed conventions to determine the derivation of one story vis-à-vis another, or a minimyth vis-à-vis a maximyth, when both stories appear to be from the same mythic cycle. So, for example, to gauge the likely chronology of two myths with similar content, for many textual historians it has long been standard practice to read the shorter of the two, the minimyth, as the precursor to the longer, the maximyth. The reason for such a calculation is that the basic structures of a story are usually thought to have come first. Ornamentation, character development, setting details, and so forth come later. This is only a basic rule of thumb, of course, and Indian literature presents exceptions to this loose guideline, where sometimes a longer version is older and has been cut down over time.[30] Thus, while one could make the case that the longer version of "Dakṣa's Sacrifice" in the *Carakasaṃhitā*'s section on therapeutics (*cikitsāsthāna*) developed out of the shorter version situated first in the list of five minimyths above, it is difficult to posit a definitive chronology given that the narrative of "Dakṣa's Sacrifice" was already well known during the time of the development of the classical ayurvedic sources.

There are many important similarities and divergences among the five passages in which the minimyths occur. Dakṣa is mentioned directly in only two of the five minimyths, namely, the *Aṣṭāṅgahṛdayasaṃhitā* and *Mādhavanidāna*. Of the five, only the *Aṣṭāṅgahṛdayasaṃhitā* attributes fever directly to improper behavior; furthermore, it equates fever with evil and death. The minimyths in the *Carakasaṃhitā*'s Nidānasthāna and the *Suśrutasaṃhitā* link fever to karma and multiple lives. Āyurveda's great trio (*bṛhattrayī*)—the *Carakasaṃhitā*, *Suśrutasaṃhitā*, and *Aṣṭāṅgahṛdayasaṃhitā*—is unified on the claim that fever strikes individuals at birth and at death. The reference in the *Bhelasaṃhitā* is unique among the five minimyths because it puts the onus on the physician, not the patient, to placate Maheśvara in order to treat fever. The reference to Maheśvara almost reads like an afterthought in *Bhela*, in that fever is not the progeny of Rudra or Śiva but a fierce aspect (*raudra*) of Maheśvara.[31] Finally, the *Mādhavanidāna* passage is noteworthy for the fact that it is little more than the minimyth itself. This text, from the eighth century C.E., also presents us with perhaps a very old remnant of the original fever minimyth or, conversely, a terrific example of a story potentially shortening, rather than lengthening, over time.

Returning to the maximyth in the *Carakasaṃhitā*'s Cikitsāsthāna, what does the story tell us about the origins and consequences of fever? What does the story reveal about the perceptions of the story's authors about the links between human biology, society, and religion? Two important elements about fever jump out straightaway in the story's opening two lines. Fever, the text says, is a consequence of attachment (*parigraha*). The next line (the minimyth) states that the source of fever is Rudra's anger. These two statements do not fit together tidily. They do not entirely contradict each other, but their syntactic relation is odd. These two lines, I suggest, are two segments of a four-part inference intimated in the narrative as we have it: the second premise and a conclusion (*b* and *d* shown in the list below). Unsaid, though clearly understood, as we shall see once we look into the intertextual referencing in the story, are the first and third premises (*a* and *c*), which would read: "attachment arose among human beings due to a cosmic decline in dharma" and "dharmic decline makes Rudra angry." Taken together, the complete formation would read:

a. Attachment arose due to a cosmic decline in dharma

b. Fever is a consequence of attachment

c. Dharmic decline makes Rudra angry

d. Fever arises out of Rudra's anger

I hasten to point out that I am not proposing the authors or redactors of this classical medical work did not or could not properly formulate an inferential statement. Rather, I contend that the opening verse of the medical adaptation of "Dakṣa's Sacrifice" in the *Carakasaṃhita* is a combination of two minimyths, one about fever arising out of Rudra's anger and another about fever arising on account of attachment. On my reading, what I have called the missing first and third premises in fact unfold in the course of the narrative. They are the narrative accoutrements that transform the two minimyths into a single maximyth. To understand their relationship, we must explore the history of fever in Sanskrit literature and medicine, a history that was certainly available and known to audiences of the classical Sanskrit medical sources in premodern India but perhaps is not so readily identifiable to audiences today. In the remainder of this chapter I explore the history of fever in Indian medical literature, and I address the two minimyths in the Dakṣa story—the association of fever with attachment and with Rudra's anger—in view of each story's relation to Hindu cosmology and the complex religious principles of dharma and karma.

Fever in Brief Historical Outline

The Sanskrit noun *jvara* occurs in the *Atharvaveda* in the compound *aṅgajvara*, "body fever," possibly referring to a kind of lymphadenitis.[32] Conventional practice in the history of Indian medicine has been to connect the term *jvara* with a disease in the *Atharvaveda* called *takmán*. Jean Filliozat speculated that the Atharvavedic term *takmán* survived as the term *ātaṅka*, "pain or disease in the body," in the classical ayurvedic compendium of Caraka and in Vāgbhaṭa's *Aṣṭāṅgahṛdayasaṃhitā*.[33] Filliozat's argument, however, appears to rest on "a certain assonance" he recognized between the words *takmán* and *ātaṅka*.[34] Although I agree with Filliozat that there is a historical relationship between the two words, the relationship appears to be more contingent on differing semantic determiners (in English these are prefixes and suffixes) that have been affixed to a single root rather than accented vocalic rhyming. In later classical Sanskrit literature, *ātaṅka* is synonymous with *jvara* and the bodily pain a person experiences from the disease. This is the case in medical literature, as Filliozat rightly noticed, as well as in non-medical literature, as we find, for example, in the *Yājñavalkyasmṛti* and Kālidāsa's *Abhijñānaśākuntalam*.[35] The reason for the historical relationship is based on the standard derivation of both the Atharvavedic *takmán* and the classical Sanskrit *ātaṅka* from the verbal root √tañc, "to contract, shrink; to coagulate." The connection of this verbal root with fever, or even with an elevation of heat in general, might seem counterintuitive, for the application or presence of heat typically expands or bloats most substances, whereas the application of cold shrinks them. This is certainly true in most instances. It is also the case, however, that an elemental form of heat like fire reduces substances to nothing, in effect shrinking them in the extreme. What is more, in terms of human physiology, feverish human bodies tend to become dehydrated, which characteristically produces at least the appearance of a shrinking or attenuation of the body. To map out the linguistic relationship between *takmán* and *ātaṅka* from the Vedic to the classical period and even later, one would have to follow the changing use of the root √tañc and its derivatives, a task well beyond the scope of this book. Instead, I wish to offer a brief survey of the historical representation and literary figuration of fever in Sanskrit literature.

The symptoms of *takmán* in the *Atharvaveda* are similar to two types of fever in Caraka's compendium called seasonal and intermittent fevers.[36] Kenneth Zysk has shown, however, that descriptions of *takmán* in the *Atharvaveda* imply that there are more than a few types of fever whose characteristics include chills and a high body temperature.[37] In terms of pathology, the *Atharvaveda* provides little to no information regarding *takmán*. Its cause, and the very disease itself, are imagined in the text as a divine force that enters and in some way distresses a victim's body and thereby produces illness. Routine associations in the *Atharvaveda* with prominent Vedic deities such as Rudra appear to have had an apotheosis-effect on *takmán*, and it thus became divine by association.[38] Worshippers invoke the god Takman by the name Hrūḍu; he is said to originate from the god of fire, Agni; he is called the son of Varuṇa, and he is routinely linked to the god Rudra.[39] Metaphors for fever in the *Atharvaveda* include thunderbolts (*vajras*) and Rudra's missiles (*hetis*), both of which are said to strike victims swiftly and without warning, but usually during the monsoon season.[40] Other diseases in fever's Vedic family include a brother, swelling (*balāsa*), a sister, cough (*kāsikā*), and a cousin, dermatitis (*pāman*).[41]

During the Vedic period, diseases were often identified with environmental forces. Observation and experience revealed to the Vedic sages that human bodies undergo changes in step with the seasons. In most parts of South Asia, the monsoon has always ushered in the most severe climatic transformation of the calendar year. Severe humidity and dampness, both of which lead to a proliferation of malaria-bearing mosquitoes, and extensive temperature fluctuations during the monsoon season tend to elevate the number of ailments that typically do not arise in the hot and dry seasons among human populations. A full-fledged understanding of the interior of a human body (that is, anything resembling what today we would call anatomy) is absent in Sanskrit literature before the classical period, when the *Suśrutasaṃhitā* presents us with the most thoroughgoing account of the parts of the body and their relationships to one another. Apart from afflictions clearly caused by sources external to oneself (such as an arm cut by a knife or a nose struck by a fist), the composers of the *Atharvaveda* regularly attributed the occurrence of an illness apparently originating in the interior of the body, such as fever, to divine malevolence.[42]

Therefore, to treat a disease, the Vedic healer (*bhiṣaj*) had to attend to the disease-deity associated with the disorder. In the case of fever, the disease-deity was Takman. The healer's task was not to annihilate Takman entirely. Rather, Takman's grip on the feverish victim's body would first be loosened through religious rituals, the recitation of mantras, and the ingestion of botanical decoctions.[43] Then the healer would relocate Takman to wherever he was thought to have come from, or the healer would simply attempt to move him to any place other than the patient's body.[44] Often the *Atharvaveda* recommends that a healer transfer a disease-deity to the bodies of certain animals—to a parakeet (*śuka*) in the case of jaundice, for example, because its yellowish color was thought to absorb jaundice and carry it far away from the afflicted, or to a frog (*maṇḍūka*) in case of fever, because its cool and wet body was supposed to neutralize the powerful heat of fever.[45] Otherwise a Vedic healer might lay a disease-deity to rest somewhere it would be unlikely to inflict more harm, such as deep within the ground.[46] To treat fever in the human body, the *Bhelasaṃhitā*, a Sanskrit medical source coeval to, and according to some older than, the *Carakasaṃhitā*, echoes the advice of the *Atharvaveda* to appease the god—in *Bhela* the god is an irate Śiva—from whom fever comes.[47]

The relocation, rather than annihilation of something that is harmful to oneself, or something that one naturally does not want involved in one's life, such as any evil being, is a common motif in Hindu mythology. Diseases in the narratives of Sanskrit medical literature often appear much like evil entities in this regard. As we saw, the minimyth of Rudra's anger in the *Aṣṭāṅgahṛdayasaṃhitā* flatly equates fever with evil. Wendy Doniger O'Flaherty has shown that the ancient Indian conception of evil, *pāpa*, carries a dual sense, in that it may signify the opposite of both physical and ethical goodness. Furthermore, *pāpa* may signify two discernibly different types of evil, which O'Flaherty calls "ethical evils" and "natural evils." Ethical evils are horrible acts that humans perform, such as murder and burglary; natural evils are terrible things or events that, for the most part, arise without direct human influence, such as tsunamis, hurricanes, and some diseases.[48] This distinction is obvious in the Sanskrit language at the time of the *Atharvaveda*. The occurrence of *takmán* in a human being is, by and large, not the result of an ethical evil that a person commits. Fever is evil not in the ethical sense of what one does; rather, it is a natural evil. Following O'Flaherty, fever "is [something] we do not wish to have done to us."[49] In the *Atharvaveda*, fever is malevolence born utterly of nonhuman causes.

The *Carakasaṃhitā* maintains the Vedic understanding of fever as a natural evil, or natural disease, but only up to a point. In its longer narrative of fever in the Cikitsāsthāna, the incidence of fever is linked by intertextual reference to a natural decline in dharma that accompanies the cosmic calendar. The origin of fever in the human world is intimately tied to the socioreligious lapse inherent in the dénouement of the First Cosmic Age. There are natural causes (or natural evils) common to all people, occurring at the moments of birth and death, a view also expressed in the shorter of the two fever narratives in the *Carakasaṃhitā*, namely, the account in the section on pathology (*nidānasthāna*). The ethical cause (or ethical evil) is mapped out in the narrative according to the actions of an archetypal patient, Dakṣa-Prajāpati.[50] Fever occurs as a transference of painful heat. The painful heat initially transfers from Rudra to Dakṣa on account of Dakṣa's dharmically reprehensible behavior. But after having established the actions of Dakṣa as the model against whom to judge the propriety of socioreligious behavior, Rudra declares that the child born of his rage should exist as fever in the world at the three times of birth, death, and among people acting reprehensibly. Rudra remains the source of fever in all cases, whether natural or ethical. Before we can make sense of the centrality of Rudra to the narrative of fever in the medical context, the minimyth of fever and attachment must be explored.

Fever and Attachment

Apart from the initial reference, the word "attachment" (*parigraha*) does not appear again in the fever narrative. The clue to interpret its meaning is in the first section of the second verse, which states that Rudra took a vow of non-anger for 1,000 divine years in the Second Age, the Tretā Yuga, of Hinduism's cyclical calendar of Four Cosmic Ages (*yugas*).[51] The timing of Rudra's vow is significant, and someone familiar with the *Carakasaṃhitā* in the form in which we have it today would know that in the text's section on measures (*vimānasthāna*) there is a rather telling story about the cycle of cosmic ages and the occurrence of disease among humankind. According to this story, during the First Cosmic Age, the Satya (or Kṛta) Yuga, very rarely did bad things happen.[52] When bad things began to occur, the text explains, humankind's lack of dharma, or neglect of social and religious duty, was the cause.[53] From one cosmic age to the next, the universal bank of dharma is said to decrease by one-fourth. The cosmos undergoes a long, slow, and steady deterioration from the First Age to the Fourth Age, from the Satya Yuga to the Kali Yuga, until a final dissolution (*pralaya*) occurs, after which the cycle starts anew with the first and most pleasurable age. All of the degradations that occur in the universe both are caused by flagging dharma and in turn bring about conditions that encourage people to neglect their dharma.

At the close of the First Age and the start of the Second Age, when Rudra was in the midst of his vow of non-anger, human dharma began to disintegrate because of people's gluttonous behavior. Gluttony consequently caused peoples' bodies to become heavy; their heaviness gave way to fatigue; fatigue led to carelessness, which in turn generated attachment to, and the accumulation of, material things. Attachment and accumulation bred ownership, and ownership bred greed; greed gave way to duplicity, anger, violence, and grief. Attendant deprivations in nature occurred: there was one-fourth less rainfall in each descending age, causing the earth's vitality to diminish by one-fourth from age to age. This in turn caused an equal plummet in the nutrient levels of food. People's diets thus suffered, and the integrity of their bodies weakened. As a result, diseases easily invaded human bodies.[54] Curiously, in the Second Cosmic Age religious practices blossomed, especially ritual sacrifices, despite the fact that dharma declined universally. The reason for this, following the explanation of the commentator Cakrapāṇidatta, was that the objectives motivating people to sacrifice were not honorable; people did not sacrifice out of a sense of dharmic obligation, but rather out of attachment to and desire for material gain.[55]

The lessening of dharma alongside the descending and deleterious cosmic ages is central to the explanation in the *Carakasaṃhitā* of how fever found its way into the world and into human bodies. The illustration of Dakṣa and his sacrificial neglect conveys the message that fever is a biophysical condition born of certain improvident and immoral modes of being human in the world. The word "attachment" (*parigraha*) serves as a master-metonym denoting all non-dharmic human qualities like greed, violence, lethargy, duplicity, and so on, while the Dakṣa character neatly stands in as a metaphor for the paradigmatic, dharmically unsound patient. His non-dharmic qualities challenge the Hindu notion of "common *dharma*" (*sāmānyadharma*)—those things that all people are obliged to do at all times to maintain operational societies and civilizations. The association between fever and attachment here is anchored in the theory of cyclically descending cosmic ages. As the ages go by, everything naturally falls apart, including socioreligious duties and human uprightness, both moral and biophysical. What is more, vital to Hinduism's theory of descending cosmic ages is the idea that for the cycle to complete itself and start anew, certain weaknesses and failings must arise before others. From earlier failings and weaknesses more failings and weaknesses in the human world are born, and so on. Following the logic of the cosmic history of disease in general and Rudra's actions in the fever narrative, fever appears to be understood as a biophysical condition born of certain morally and mentally digressive states of human activity in the world, described in the *Carakasaṃhitā* as adharmic behavior.

The view that a lack of dharma was significant to the dissolution and ensuing reconstitution of the universe, and significant to classical Indian cosmography generally, bespeaks an intellectual attitude concerning the structure of the universe and history during the time of the compilation of the text attributed to Caraka. The medical rendition of the Four Cosmic Ages offered here does not accord with most Hindu astronomers of the day, however, who generally pointed to orbital decline among the planets as the causal force propelling the progression of the cosmic ages. The astronomer's calculation of time (*kāla*) in the model of Four Cosmic Ages, as Romila Thapar has suggested, was for the most part based on logical positivistic suppositions that were supposed to be falsifiable.[56] The view in the *Carakasaṃhitā* that the grand cosmic cycle (*mahāyuga*) is simultaneously a result and a source of non-dharma (*adharma*) resembles cosmological theories that were unfolding and fast becoming popular in non-astronomical sources in the early centuries of the Common Era, such as those contained in *The Laws of Manu*, the *Mahābhārata*, and the Purāṇas.[57]

The compilers of the classical Sanskrit medical literature worked from an expansive "disciplinary" worldview by today's standards; for them, modern cultural domains that are regularly seen as antinomic today, such as science and religion, were clearly not regarded as incongruous in the elaboration of knowledge that leads to long life (*āyurveda*). Given the rather exhaustive coverage of the classical medical compendia, it is hardly extraordinary to find in these texts routine usage and reinterpretation of concepts and practices found in other areas of Sanskrit knowledge systems that are more religious, philosophical, sociological, and cosmological than medical. The foregoing example from the field of astronomy is indeed just a fraction of the interplay between Indian medicine and astronomy. The section on the sense organs (*indriyasthāna*) in the *Carakasaṃhitā*, for example, contains a wealth of information on the uses of omens and the planets in determining health and treating illness. Later Sanskrit medical treatises expand on this material in the compendium of Caraka. The fourteenth-century *Vīrasiṃhāvalokaḥ*, which draws elaborate correlations between the human body and the constellations, is an excellent example of this integrative medicine. Long life requires somatic lessons of all sorts, of course, and whether they are in typical chart talk or narrative form, the knowledge of the Sanskrit medical literature aspires to a holistic consideration of the human body's potential productiveness and damage in society and the larger world. The narratives of Āyurveda use the gods as models to elaborate this. They are well-known stories, as "Dakṣa's Sacrifice" would have been in classical India. They also lend themselves well to multiple interpretations and uses, which is why we speak of "cycles" of mythic narratives across many genres of Sanskrit literature, for many versions of the stories of the lives of the gods and goddesses appear in diverse literary contexts. To round out our understanding of the ways in which a common somatic disorder like fever developed in the imaginations of the compilers of Indian medicine, we need to look at the earliest historical records of fever in Vedic literature, which connect the god Rudra to a biophysical ailment. The historical data are especially important to establish why the authors of the text might have decided to use a narrative involving Rudra in particular to explain the physical disorder of fever.

Fever and Rudra's Anger

What made the god Rudra so upset? How can we explain the etiology of fever tied to Rudra's violent reaction to the dharmic failings that occur around him in the narrative of "Dakṣa's Sacrifice"? When the cosmos undergoes a shift from the First Cosmic Age to the Second Cosmic Age, the human world was stumbling into a state lacking dharma; meanwhile, Rudra was attending to his vow of non-anger (*akrodhavrata*). We have already seen the cosmic and environmental connections between dharma and fever, which the compilers of the *Carakasaṃhitā* carefully linked through intertextual references. To make sense of the god Rudra in this narrative and his relationship to fever, the cosmic decline in dharma in relation to religious practice is important. There are two aspects of the narrative that nicely represent a classical medical commentary on, and reinterpretation of, important religious concepts in Hinduism: vow-taking and the dharma of a sacrificer.

It is quite out of character for Rudra to play the role of a peacenik in Hindu mythology. He is usually a pugnacious godly bruiser. When it comes to medical or healing activity, he is prone to passive-aggressive behavior, as Palmyr Cordier observed in his doctoral study of ancient Indian medicine, citing the Vedicist Abel Bergaigne: "Rudra is a terrible and feared doctor. 'He strikes as he heals,' explained A. Bergaigne, 'and repairs those evils that he has caused.' "[58] And yet in the narrative encounter of Dakṣa and Rudra in the *Carakasaṃhitā*, Rudra is engaged in a vow of non-anger for 1,000 divine years (or what amounts to 360,000 human years). In Hinduism, vows often involve the observance of great physical and mental restrictions, such as fasting, celibacy, and meditation, among other things. The idea is that through great sacrifice a vow taker will sublimate the qualities that he or she has forsaken into a special, perhaps supernatural, power, such as the power of flight, the ability to be in multiple places at one time, the power to restore health, and so forth. For humans, the basic idea behind the vow is that great sacrifice will attract the attention of the gods, who will grace the human vow taker with a boon, be it be material, mental, or mystical (e.g., cows, an excellent memory, or *mokṣa*). In Hindu mythology, gods, goddesses, demons, and great sages also often take vows, and they take them for many of the same reasons that humans do. I have not come across another example in the Sanskrit literature in which Rudra undertakes a vow of non-anger like the one we find in the compendium of Caraka. Rudra's abstinence from anger, however, reads very much like an analogue to the abstinence from sexual activity of the god Śiva, who as we have seen is regularly taken to be a direct mythological descendant of Rudra in the Hindu pantheon. In numerous Hindu myths, the energy Śiva accumulates from celibacy provides him with the ability to engage in extended sexual activity.[59] Whereas the abnegation of sex leads to periods of enormous sexual constancy for Śiva, for Rudra the denial of anger for 1,000 divine years culminates is a storm of fury, which he let loose on the demons, Dakṣa, and Dakṣa's sacrificial grounds and attendants.

The longer of the two fever narratives in the *Carakasaṃhitā*, the Cikitsāsthāna version, does not tell us Rudra's original intent for taking his vow, so we do not know how, when, or why (or even if) he intended to apply the sublimated energy he accumulated during his vow. The story does tell us that his vow spanned a great length of time and that it included the practice of religious austerities and the accumulation of great "heat"—*tapas*, which refers to both the religious practice and the internal heat accumulated from the practice. By entirely suspending anger during his vow, Rudra caused a great deal of *tapas* to well up inside himself, and that heat in turn gave him great power. Although the story does not expressly reveal Rudra's original aim for taking the vow of non-anger, the text does tell us that someone upset Rudra so severely that he decided to unleash the heat he amassed on that person when his vow ended.

Rudra's pent-up anger is directed toward Dakṣa, and for two reasons. The first reason speaks directly to the chief aim of classical Āyurveda—to ensure long life (*āyus*) by providing people with knowledge (*veda*) about how to live optimally according to their mental and physical abilities. In Sanskrit, the name Dakṣa means "able" and "intelligent." It is understood, therefore, that Dakṣa was both aware and capable of quashing the demons that disturbed Rudra while he was committed to his vow of pacifism. Yet Dakṣa did nothing. The second reason pertains to religious practice. Dakṣa prepared a sacrifice (*yajña*) to which he invited all of the gods, offering each god a proper share of the ritual oblations. But Dakṣa did not invite Rudra. This omission, the gods warned Dakṣa, would render the sacrifice an utter failure and create bedlam at the sacrificial grounds. Indeed, Dakṣa's deliberate sacrificial insolence so insulted Rudra, that at the close of his vow he became irate. He shot a fire-child through the air out of the inferno streaming from his third eye, and that child proceeded to destroy Dakṣa's sacrifice. When Rudra leveled Dakṣa's sacrifice, everyone attending experienced the sensation of being aflame (presumably Dakṣa-Prajāpati did as well, although he conspicuously is not mentioned by name). The mass sensation of fever here intimates a notion of contagion that percolates beneath the surface story, especially in connection with large-scale epidemic-type illnesses. The immediate source of the infectious contamination, echoing the cosmic spiral into *adharma* seen in the above theory of the cosmic ages, is a morally corrupt actor whose failure to uphold his dharmic duties at the sacrifice led to disease and an outbreak among the people near him.[60] The vector of fever is the unnamed anger-child, who in non-medical versions of this story is frequently known as the fearsome god Vīrabhadra. The people affected as a result of Dakṣa's actions are rendered guilty (or ill) by association.

It is not clear from the *Carakasaṃhitā*'s rendition of this story why Dakṣa did not invite Rudra to the sacrifice. The relationship between Rudra and Dakṣa-Prajāpati has a long history in Sanskrit literature that offers several pieces of the foundation on which the medical variant of the narrative of fever was clearly based. The central part of the Dakṣa story goes back to the *Ṛgveda* and its commentarial literature, the Brāhmaṇas, where Prajāpati commits incest with his "irresistible young daughter," Uṣas.[61] Two later Vedic commentaries, the *Śatapatha Brāhmaṇa* and *Aitareya Brāhmaṇa,* expand the Ṛgvedic account along the following story line: Prajāpati's sons, the gods, are shocked by their father's incestuous act with their sister, and so they urge Rudra to slay Prajāpati with an arrow. Rudra fires his arrow, and it strikes Prajāpati. As Prajāpati's dying body slumped, some of his semen fell to the ground. Because Prajāpati symbolizes the primordial sacrifice of creation itself, every part of his dying body had to be offered as part of the sacrifice, including his semen. The gods took his semen to the god Bhaga, who protects the southern end of the Vedic sacrificial ground. Upon looking at the semen, Bhaga's eyes burned up, and he became blind. The gods then took the semen to Pūṣan, the all-seeing solar deity and patron of journeys; he tasted it and his teeth immediately fell out.[62]

Another Brāhmaṇa, the *Gopatha Brāhmaṇa,* basically relates the same story regarding Bhaga's blindness and Pūṣan's loss of teeth. The confrontation between Prajāpati and Rudra, however, which results in Prajāpati spilling his seed, differs from the accounts in the *Śatapatha* and *Aitareya Brāhmaṇas* and instead depicts a clash between the two deities, Prajāpati and Rudra, which is strikingly akin to the medical narrative in the compendium of Caraka. The *Gopatha Brāhmaṇa*'s account centers on a sacrifice that Prajāpati prepares, sometimes called the "Prāśitra Story": Prajāpati defies Rudra by refusing to offer him a share of the sacrifice. Violently upset, Rudra helps himself to a portion of the sacrifice, the so-called *prāśitra*-food, and then presents the *prāśitra* to the divinities who maintain the sacrificial grounds. Its mere presence wreaks physical troubles on nearly all of them. By turns, it is given to Bhaga, whom it blinds; to Savitṛ, whom it makes handless (then golden-handed); to Pūṣan, whom it makes toothless; to Idhma Āṅgirasa, whom it beheads; to Varhi, whose body's joints become dislocated; and lastly to Bṛhaspati Āṅgirasa, who uses his expertise with mantras to render the *prāśitra* innocuous.[63]

In these early versions of "Dakṣa's Sacrifice," as in the compendium of Caraka, Rudra does not kill Dakṣa. In a non-medical and chronologically later version than the Vedic stories, the *Mahābhārata* epic contains an account of "Dakṣa's Sacrifice" that is analogous (and relatively coeval) to the *Carakasaṃhitā*. The story of Rudra's destruction of Dakṣa's sacrifice (*dakṣayajñanāśa*) in the *Mahābhārata* takes place in the context of the marriage of Śiva and Umā. When the Lord of Creatures, Dakṣa-Prajāpati, prepares a great sacrifice and does not offer oblations to Śiva, Umā draws attention to this disrespect for her partner, impelling Śiva to destroy Dakṣa's sacrificial grounds. Umā is one of Śiva's many wives, but in the *Mahābhārata* she is not said to be Dakṣa's daughter, and there are no allusions to the incestuous element of the story found in the Vedas and Brāhmaṇas.[64]

In Kālidāsa's *Kumārasambhava* and in some of the Purāṇas, the father-daughter relationship between Dakṣa and Satī, who is one of Śiva's wives, is clear. The Purāṇas and *Kumārasambhava* appear to have merged the Vedic and epic developments into a single myth about Śiva and Satī. Rudra punishes Dakṣa-Prajāpati for his incestuous act with Uṣas, and Rudra (or Śiva) punishes Dakṣa-Prajāpati for excluding him from the sacrifice.[65] In these stories, Dakṣa-Prajāpati performs a large sacrifice, to which he invited neither his daughter, Satī, nor his son-in-law, Śiva. We learn in the Purāṇic accounts that Dakṣa, resembling fathers the world over, is not pleased with his daughter's choice of a mate, the dreadlocked, ash-covered, cremation-ground-meditating Śiva.[66] Although she was uninvited, Satī drops in unannounced at her father's sacrifice. Upon her arrival, her father publicly insults her, which greatly upsets Satī, and, in Kālidāsa's account, Satī immolates herself on the sacrificial fire her father had prepared.[67] When Śiva receives the news of Satī's death he becomes enraged, races to the site where Satī died, and violently destroys Dakṣa's sacrifice. By some accounts, Śiva beheads Dakṣa, and in other versions Śiva creates a violent demon named Vīrabhadra, who destroys the sacrifice and beheads Dakṣa.[68] In most versions of the story, Śiva revives Dakṣa after killing him, gives him the head of a goat, and restores the sacrifice, after which Dakṣa openly praises Śiva as the supreme deity (*parameśvara*).

In medieval recensions of the Dakṣa story, after learning of Satī's self-immolation, Śiva destroys Dakṣa's sacrifice. Thereafter he becomes so brokenhearted that he sweeps up Satī's dead body, slings her over his shoulder, and sadly roams the earth. To rid Śiva of his terrible grief, in some versions of the story, the gods enter into Satī's dead body and disassemble it bit by bit. Each location a piece of her body fell to the ground later becomes commemorated as a sacred pilgrimage site (*pīṭha*, literally "seat"), of which there are fifty-one scattered across the South Asian landscape.[69]

Returning to the Dakṣa story in the *Carakasaṃhitā*, we see that it is the gods and sages who calm Rudra down with songs of praise. This makes Rudra *śiva*, "auspicious." The child born of Rudra's anger then asks what he should do next for his father. It is at this point that we first encounter the Sanskrit term for "fever," *jvara*, in the narrative. The great length of Rudra's vow, whether or not it was his intent, resulted in the production of fever. The fact that Rudra's vow involved the containment of anger, his natural temperament, highlights the austerity of his undertaking, and thus the great power he accumulated from it, and starkly contrasts with the carelessness of Dakṣa's religious practice. In response to his child's question about his future role among humanity, Rudra explains that the child, literally his "angerfire" (*krodhāgni*), should afflict human beings with fever at two fixed and inevitable stages of life and in the event of a probable, though avertable, third instance: at birth, at death, and when people act reprehensively.

Rudra's injunction to his offspring nicely captures a common trope in Sanskrit medical narratives that at the end of the day, all people fall under the rubric of "patient," not simply because human bodies are susceptible to disease, which they naturally are, but because every person experiences the psychosocial experience of illness. Every person will be a patient, and because actions and decisions play a substantial role in health, every thinking and acting person is accountable for the illnesses he or she experiences. These stories merely help to identify where one might have gone wrong given the sickness that manifests. This is addressed by the third instance in which Rudra's angerfire should become fever among humanity—in cases of improper behavior. Dakṣa commits an improper act (*apacāra*) by not inviting Rudra to attend his sacrifice. His dharma as a sacrificer is to entreat the gods. Because he does not appease Rudra by fixing the god a share of his sacrificial offerings, Dakṣa exposes himself as well as those around him to the malady of fever. Of the three instances in which Rudra's offspring should manifest as fever, improper behavior is the most crucial for the compilers of the this medical text, I would argue. This cause applies to everyday dharmic behavior that, more often than not, people can attend to and actually adjust in their lives. Fever is the direct fruit of karma, or one's actions, and it is explicitly tied to knowledge in this case. When one's karma produces illness, often the cause is a violation or misuse of knowledge (*prajñāparādha*).[70] Violations of knowledge involve activities marked by an erroneous or faulty sense of judgment. I have already explained that Dakṣa violates his knowledge as a sacrificer; likewise, though he was aware of and presumably able to ward off the demons that pestered Rudra while he was undertaking his vow of non-anger, Dakṣa did nothing. Unlike other Sanskrit medical sources, such as the *Aṣṭāṅgahṛdayasaṃhitā* and the *Suśrutasaṃhitā*, which tend to interpret the concept of karma as the fuel that drives saṃsāric rebirth and redeath, the authors of the *Carakasaṃhitā*, as Mitchell Weiss has noted, "in effect redefined the concept of *karma*, shifting the emphasis from past lives to present behavior in such a way to make it clinically germane."[71] In the medical context of Caraka's compendium the story of "Dakṣa's Sacrifice" is about a person's karmic imprint in the current moment and the repercussions of that imprint in a person's current lifetime. Karmic fruit reveals an aptitude to act properly or not act properly. Who determines the parameters of proper behavior? In this case the draftsmen of the text did. They appropriated a popular ritual narrative to their medical agenda, deciding what should be considered right and wrong, good and bad, and so forth, drawing from the social-moral-legal sources of the Dharmaśāstra literature and the six Hindu philosophical schools (*ṣaḍdarśana*), especially Sāṃkhya and Vaiśeṣika.

In the verse immediately following the Dakṣa narrative, the *Carakasaṃhitā* states that the occurrence of fever in one's lifetime manifests in heat, aversion to food, thirst, lethargy, and heart pain. But at birth and death, fever manifests in the form of *tamas*.[72] Why *tamas*? The primary meaning of *tamas* is "darkness," and here it refers to its metaphorical sense of ignorance. To make sense of the way in which *tamas* is used in the fever narrative, embryological passages in a non-medical text, the *Mārkaṇḍeya Purāṇa*, are useful.[73] In this text, the gestating fetus is fully aware of his or her previous births, and mindful of every deed and misdeed committed over countless lifetimes, the fetus knows what to do upon delivery to erase the karmic residue that has built up from birth to birth. The period of gestation appears to be so pleasant in this text that the fetus laments his impending departure from the womb.[74] The *Mārkaṇḍeya Purāṇa* continues, in all likelihood following the much earlier *Garbha Upaniṣad*, to explain that at the time a child exits the womb, the "illusion of Viṣṇu" (*vaiṣṇavīmāyā*) sweeps over the newborn and erases all memories, good and bad, of past lives.[75] In the *Carakasaṃhitā* it appears that fever has a function similar to Viṣṇu's illusion. Elsewhere in this medical text there is a reference to the "wind of delivery" (*prasūtimāruta*), though the effect of this wind on a newborn at the moment of delivery is not offered.[76] Minoru Hara has written about a phenomenon that causes the loss of memory of previous lives at birth known as *janmaduḥkha*, "suffering of birth." It is the suffering of birth, Hara writes, from entering the world covered in feces and amniotic fluid, from having been squeezed through a narrow passageway, "that is responsible for the loss of memory (*smṛti*) and knowledge (*vijñāna*), which the ordinary human being in the state of embryo is supposed to possess until the last moment of his stay in his mother's womb."[77] In the medical narrative of fever in the *Carakasaṃhitā*, a parallel story of traumatic life beginnings is suggested in the manifestation of *tamas* in the form of a fever at the moment of birth, which induces a kind of amnesia-inducing darkness in a newborn. This darkness effectively nullifies the newborn's capacity to ensure that mistakes of past lives will not be repeated in his or her brand new life. Because fever also strikes all humans at the moment of death with the same *tamas* experienced at birth, the authors of the *Carakasaṃhitā* leave room neither for the remembrance of things done in past lives nor for the strategizing about what to do in the next life like the fetus has occasion to do in the *Mārkaṇḍeya Purāṇa*.

Why would the classical medical authors make this move? By framing human life with fever at birth and death, they underscore the empirical and practical significance of people's actions in their present lives. For all people, physiologic well-being depends on more than hygiene, diet, and exercise. As Āyurveda's medical narratives demonstrate, what is good for oneself also depends on the ways in which one acts according to one's abilities and performs one's socioreligious responsibilities. In other words, storytelling about fever in the Sanskrit medical literature, as the somatic lessons of the miscarriage and king's disease narratives in the next two chapters also show, suggest that health is at once a product of a person's karma and dharma and a precondition for the performance of sound socioreligious activity.

Chapter 4

Miscarriage

To what extent do we control the ways we use our bodies when we act in the world? Are our actions deliberate? Do we act with complete and mindful intention? Or are our actions products of an ever-present social programming, an "education of movements," as Marcel Mauss famously called it, that is impressed upon us from other people, cultural institutions, and social forces?[1] In this chapter, I investigate these questions of intention and thoughtful action through an analysis of the role of narrative in the development of knowledge about, and rationalization for, conditioning the human body in a medical compendium devoted to women's and children's health, the *Kāśyapasaṃhitā*. In particular, I examine a narrative about demonic possession of women that results in the biological crisis of miscarriage. As we shall see, alongside an overt regulation of the female body, the narrative also endeavors to regulate the woman's mind. But control of the mind, I suggest, serves the larger goal of the story, which is to manage the mechanics of a woman's physical body by curtailing opportunities for her intrapersonal activity and social self-expression.

Given that miscarriage is the central event of the medical narrative discussed in this chapter, I am concerned here primarily with the *Kāśyapasaṃhitā*'s treatment of the female body, and especially the feminine power to produce offspring. The authors of the miscarriage narrative in the *Kāśyapasaṃhitā* attempt to explain what happens to the process of human reproduction when pregnant women do not stay the course of a certain socioreligious etiquette. A host of divine characters in the story serve as standard bearers of good and bad behavior for human observers to ponder. Among those models, two are central: a goddess, Revatī, and her aggressive avatar, Jātahāriṇī. Their story offers a vivid and straightforward example of the use of narrative logic to explain a somatic calamity. Beginning with an elaborate creation account, the story analogizes the physiologic functioning a woman experiences during miscarriage with hostilities that take place in the heavens among the gods and demons. Locked in battle with the goddess Revatī is an especially violent demoness, Long Tongue (Dīrghajihvī).

Although there are historical precedents and intertextual variants of many of the story's characters, some of which I discuss where they help to clarify the meaning of the story, in this chapter I am primarily concerned with the social and religious questions couched in the *Kāśyapasaṃhitā*'s narrative itself. For example, I am interested in asking why, in the classical Indian context, the subject of miscarriage might have lent itself to a narrative explanation rather than the standard chart talk of ayurvedic discourse that predominates most of this *saṃhitā*. As there are non-narrative explanations of fever, and in the next chapter there likewise are non-narrative explanations of the king's disease, there are chart talk accounts of miscarriage in the Sanskrit medical classics. As with the narrative cycles of fever and the king's disease in the medical literature, an examination of the narrative staging of miscarriage in the *Kāśyapasaṃhitā* suggests that there are some extraordinary things at stake with this medical issue. One question that must be asked to this end, for example, is what can we learn about the gender politics of the day from this medical story. To address this question and others, I frame my analysis around the following three themes: the relationship between heaven and earth, the interpretation of a woman's somatic experience of miscarriage by the story's male authors, and the negotiation of the age-old, intractable question of nature versus nurture. Before delving into the story, I offer a summary of the Sanskrit medical compendium ascribed to Kaśyapa and its historical context.

Text-Historical Framework of the *Kāśyapasaṃhitā*

The chief subjects of the *Kāśyapasaṃhitā* are gynecology, obstetrics, and pediatrics. All three of these specializations in classical Āyurveda fall under the one field of *kaumārabhṛtya*, literally "support of the young." In this translation, the "the young" at once refers to children—thus, this medical specialization also includes pediatrics—as well as first-time and soon-to-be mothers.[2] Other similar medical classifications used in the literature in addition to *kaumārabhṛtya* include *bālacikitsā*, "the treatment of children," and *kaumāratantra*, "treatise on children." The *Kāśyapasaṃhitā* is the only currently available classical Sanskrit medical compendium that specializes entirely in the *kaumārabhṛtya* branch of ayurvedic medicine.[3]

Structurally and thematically, in the corpus of Sanskrit medical literature, the source attributed to Kaśyapa most closely corresponds to the *Carakasaṃhitā* and *Bhelasaṃhitā*.[4] Similar to the works attributed to Caraka and Bhela, for example, Kaśyapa's compendium states that it initially contained 120 chapters, which were spread over eight sections. It also has a supplementary section, or epilogue (*khilasthāna*), which is not found in the *Carakasaṃhitā* and the *Bhelasaṃhitā*. The Khilasthāna has an additional eighty chapters, which brings the total number of chapters in the text to 200. Not all of this material is available today, however. Only seventy-eight chapters have survived to the present, and almost half of these are only partially useable because of irreversible damage to the manuscripts.[5]

Although there is general agreement among historians of Indian medicine that the *Kāśyapasaṃhitā* was produced in the late classical period, at times the text presents language that appears much older than the classical era. G. Jan Meulenbeld has noted the incidence of very old Sanskrit vocabulary and phraseology in the compendium.[6] Dominik Wujastyk also has pointed out the archaic nature of the language in the *Kāśyapasaṃhitā*, which, he writes, is "otherwise known only from the Brāhmaṇas and Vedas."[7] References to certain deities, such as Prajāpati, Agni, and Soma, as well Vedic rituals (e.g., *mārutiṣṭi*) and mantras (e.g., the Soma Pavana and Sāvitṛ mantras), are among the many signs of preclassical Sanskrit language in the text. That being said, these archaisms account for only a small portion of the *Kāśyapasaṃhitā*. All things told, it is likely that the Sanskrit source available for use today underwent its final redaction at about the same time as the *Aṣṭāṅgahṛdayasaṃhitā* of Vāgbhaṭa, which places it at approximately the sixth to seventh centuries C.E.

The *Kāśyapasaṃhitā* is notable among the Sanskrit medical classics because of its specialty in *kaumārabhṛtya*. Yet it was relatively unknown in India and the West until the end of the nineteenth century. In Nepal in 1898, Haraprasad Shastri reportedly discovered one of two existing manuscripts of the *Kāśyapasaṃhitā*, although he would soon thereafter lose it. The contents of the manuscript resurfaced in Europe because Palmyr Cordier, the prodigious French Indologist and historian of Indian medicine, had made a copy of Shastri's manuscript and donated a reprographed version of his own copy to the Bibliothèque nationale de France in Paris.[8] Thirty years after Shastri's discovery in Nepal, in 1938, Hemaraj Sharma obtained the second surviving manuscript of the text in India. This manuscript amounts to a woefully incomplete set of palm leaves, with approximately 236 leaves (starting at page 29 and ending at page 265), and is marred throughout by missing lines and words.[9]

The chapters of the *Kāśyapasaṃhitā* are arranged as a series of tutorials between the famous medical sage, Kaśyapa, and a young student named Vṛddhajīvaka, "Old Reviver."[10] Vṛddhajīvaka was neither an ordinary student nor a newcomer to medicine, and he was integral to the organization and transmission of the multipart knowledge that is *kaumārabhṛtya* in this work. His centrality to the composition of the Sanskrit medical source attributed to Kaśyapa is reflected in an alternate title sometimes used for the text, *Vṛddhajīvakīya Tantra*. Naturally, there is a fair amount of folklore underlying the weight given to this significant young physician-in-training, beginning with his name. The name Jīvaka, "reviver," is an appropriate name for a healer, and indeed there are a number of celebrated physicians with the name Jīvaka in the long history of Sanskrit literature and medicine in South Asia. For Kaśyapa's student, the adjective *vṛddha* affixed to his name sets him apart from other important physicians bearing the same name. The word *vṛddha* means "old and full-grown" or "experienced and wise." It suggests that the medical knowledge of this specific Jīvaka is in some way superior to the medical knowledge of other Jīvakas known before him and in the literature, such as the two most famous, Jīvaka the pediatrician, about whom we learn in the *Bower Manuscript*, and Jīvaka Komārabhacca, the legendary Buddhist physician (incidentally, *komārabhacca* is the Pali equivalent of the Sanskrit medical term *kaumārabhṛtya*).[11]

An elaborate myth detailing the youth's mastery of ayurvedic knowledge furthermore elucidates the meaning of the name Vṛddhajīvaka. The story goes like this: Jīvaka was the son of the sage Ricīka. When he was five years old, to the disbelief and ridicule of the older sages and learned men in his village, Jīvaka began publicly expounding Kaśyapa's medical teachings. One day, while Jīvaka bathed in the Ganges River at Kanakhal, near Haridwar, he plunged into the river and emerged on the riverbank with weathered skin, a wizened brow, and a full head of gray hair. A crowd of Jīvaka's naysayers witnessed the transformation of the young boy, and immediately they accepted his medical teachings without issue, referring to him thereafter by the name Vṛddha-Jīvaka, Old Reviver. The designation of "old" signifies the experiential wisdom that comes with age, specifically with respect to the capacity to revitalize ailing bodies.[12] It is noteworthy that Kaśyapa's medical knowledge was mastered and disseminated for the first time by a child, not an erudite pupil or a seasoned physician. Because the primary focus of Kaśyapa's treatise is pediatrics and gravidity-related matters, this story can be read to suggest that, as implausible as it may seem, gestational development and childhood might be understood and explained to their fullest extents by someone who just recently experienced these stages of life. After all, as we saw in Chapter 3, there are attestations in the late-classical, early-medieval Sanskrit literary culture of embryological discussions that envision the gestating human fetus as an entirely conscious and, in many respects, fully awakened individual. On this view, one could argue that Jīvaka somehow escaped the amnesia-inducing darkness at birth described in the *Carakasaṃhitā* (or the illusion of Viṣṇu in the *Mārkaṇḍeya Purāṇa*), and therefore the memory of his own fetal development and childbirth were not wiped away when he exited his mother's womb. There are, of course, other readings. For example, of particular importance are the story's social and religious markers about the nature and perception of medical knowledge and authority in the classical period. The fact that the wise men did not believe Jīvaka when he initially expounded Kaśyapa's teachings and that they took him seriously only after he bathed in the Ganges River and, presumably, only after he appeared as they did—old, wrinkly, and gray-haired—points to the great weight placed on ritual purification (bathing in the Ganges) and many years of education (emergence from the river appearing years older) in India before a person was considered reliable or authoritative.

A mythological chain of transmission for the *Kāśyapasaṃhitā* is also given in the text, which suggests that the final redactor of Kaśyapa's dissertation on *kaumārabhṛtya* was not his student, Vṛddhajīvaka. We are told that during the Kali Yuga, Vṛddhajīvaka's version of Kaśyapa's medical teachings was lost. But this loss was temporary, for eventually a charitable demigod (*yakṣa*) named Anāyāsa recovered and preserved them. A sage in the same lineage as Vṛddhajīvaka named Vātsya acquired Anāyāsa's reproduction of Vṛddhajīvaka's rendering of Kaśyapa's teachings. Upon obtaining this, Vātsya promptly commenced a rigorous course of scholastic study and ritual austerities both to enrich his understanding of the background of the compendium's material and to prepare himself mentally and religiously to reproduce a new version of Kaśyapa's teachings to ensure a healthful future for humankind. He studied the *Ṛgveda, Yajurveda, Sāmaveda,* and their auxiliary disciplines. He amassed great *tapas* through mediation and regular sacrifices to Śiva, Kaśyapa, and the *yakṣas*. After accomplishing all of these auspicious feats, Vātsya then revised Vṛddhajīvaka's original work.[13] The version of the *Kāśyapasaṃhitā* that we have today is Vātsya's putative reproduction of Kaśyapa's teachings to Vṛddhajīvaka.

Compendium Contents

The narrative of miscarriage in the *Kāśyapasaṃhitā* is in the chapter on the ritual precepts of Revatī (*revatīkalpādhyāyaḥ*), which is one of nine chapters in the section on ritual precepts (*kalpasthāna*). Meulenbeld has pointed out that in the *Kāśyapasaṃhitā* the section on ritual precepts, unlike analogous sections on ritual precepts in the compendia ascribed to Caraka and Bhela, which deal primarily with emetics and purgative therapies, is an utter mélange of subjects.[14] The thread holding the section together is, in spite of its own vast thematic breadth, "support for the young" (*kaumārabhṛtya*).

The *Kāśyapasaṃhitā*'s narrative of miscarriage is placed in the middle of ordinary medical topics, such as botany and nutrition.[15] The first chapter of the section on ritual precepts discusses the classifications, preparations, and the mythic origin of fumigation therapy, which was gifted to human physicians from the fire god, Agni.[16] The second chapter takes up the pharmaceutical uses and legendary origin of garlic, which I translated in Chapter 1 of this volume.[17] The third chapter is about mustard oil, the best drug for treating problems of the spleen. The fourth chapter discusses six special preparations for treating eye disorders in children. The fifth chapter is about the pharmaceutical benefits of dill and wild asparagus; both of these plants are noteworthy for their promotion of fertility, lactation in postpartum mothers, virility in men, and regular menstruation. The miscarriage narrative, in the sixth chapter (*revatīkalpādhyāyaḥ*), is atypical even in the hodgepodge context of the text's section on ritual precepts. First of all, it is rather lengthy in comparison to the coverage given to other disorders in the section. But it is also unusual because of the predominance of prose in this chapter, which stands out among the widespread use of verse, or what I have been calling pithy chart talk, throughout this and the other classical medical sources. The chapter following the miscarriage narrative, the seventh chapter, is concerned with dietetics, nutrition, and medical treatments to be administered to people who have had too much or too little to eat and drink. This chapter offers a classical Indian version of what today is fashionably known as a macrobiotic diet, for it provides a list of regions in and around South Asia (including Kashmir, China, and Bactria) and matches people with foods native to their regions as a means to support digestion and overall health.[18] The eighth chapter is about so-called distinctive ritual precepts (*viśeṣakalpādhyāyaḥ*). The main topic of this chapter is a special kind of fever called "fever due to simultaneous vitiation" (*saṃnipātajvara*), which arises when two or three of the bodily humors are agitated conjointly. The ninth and final chapter of the section on ritual precepts explains the origins and the contents of the entire compendium of Kaśyapa.

Definitional Issues

Because the English term "miscarriage" has a range of literal and semantic equivalents in Sanskrit, or near equivalents, it is useful before presenting the miscarriage narrative to consider just how well the English term "miscarriage" represents the biological event that occurs in the *Kāśyapasaṃhitā*. Terms denoting miscarriage found most often in the classical and medieval Sanskrit medical literature include the following: both *garbhapāta* and *garbhacyuti*, "falling of the embryo," specifically denote a miscarriage in the later stages of pregnancy.[19] The term *garbhasrāva*, "flow or release of the embryo," indicates a miscarriage during the early stages of gestation before the embryo has taken a solid form.[20] The terms *nāgodaragarbha*, literally "serpent belly embryo," and *līnagarbha*, "sticking embryo," indicate certain types of miscarriage in which an embryo diminishes in size, becomes dry and emaciated, and eventually, if left untreated, dies.[21] The term *garbhavyāpad*, "embryo death," is the general term in Āyurveda to indicate various complications that could strike down an embryo during pregnancy.[22]

The *Kāśyapasaṃhitā* contains several discussions about the events that lead to and follow a miscarriage, but references to the specific event are rare. So, for example, Kaśyapa's compendium states that a pregnant woman may experience a "shaking of the embryo" (*garbhacyavana*), which can result in miscarriage.[23] Overeating can cause miscarriage, and some women's physiologic makeups are simply prone to produce embryos that fall to pieces.[24] The text furthermore explains that pregnant women whose bodies are not fit for bearing children have an increased chance not only of having miscarriages but also of dying during delivery.[25] The medical narrative of miscarriage that I examine below contains the *Kāśyapasaṃhitā*'s most sustained discussion of miscarriage. But, for reasons that I explain momentarily, the narrative's primary position on miscarriage tackles circumstances peripheral to the event and to a woman's direct experience of miscarriage rather than the actual event and experiences themselves.

Across the Sanskrit medical sources, eight general reasons that a woman might have a miscarriage can be found: (1) physiologic dysfunction of the pregnant woman, (2) poor exercise regimen of the pregnant woman, (3) direct trauma to a pregnant woman's abdomen, (4) psychological disorder of the pregnant woman, (5) divine influence or karmic retribution for previous actions, (6) congenital defects of the fetus, (7) abnormal positioning of the fetus in the womb, and (8) poor nutrition of the pregnant woman.[26] The narrative account of miscarriage I discuss here falls squarely under the fifth reason: divine influence or karmic retribution for a previous act. Miscarriage is portrayed as a biological failure resulting from behavioral misconduct. Biology and social agency are linked in the story through an elaborate chain of events that starts in the heavens and ends in the wombs of human and nonhuman women. The text's authors navigate several topographies in the miscarriage story before explaining what a miscarriage entails and what causes a miscarriage to occur. The story begins with the gods and the demons in the heavens, where they drum up the ethical quandary that drives the story: who should partake of the elixir of immortality? Events then take the divine and demonic cohorts racing to earth, and the narrative effectively settles in the site of greatest interest, the womb. In many ways, the womb becomes a battlefield in this story. It is the front line in a medical mêlée in which women's control of their bodies and their capacity to be in charge of their pregnancies are at stake.

The Narrative of Miscarriage

Instructing his pupil, Old Reviver (Vṛddhajīvaka), the august medical sage Kaśyapa introduces the miscarriage narrative in the following way:

> "Now we will explain the ritual precepts of Revatī."
>
> In the beginning the Lord of Creatures, Prajāpati, was alone. This is all there was. He then created Time, and he made the gods and demons, the fathers, humans, seven domestic and wild animals, medicinal plants, and the trees. As Prajāpati looked on, thereupon Hunger was born. Hunger entered Prajāpati, and he languished. So it is that hungry creatures grow weak. Soon Prajāpati noticed that the medicinal plants countered Hunger. So he ate those plants and, having digested[27] them, he was released from Hunger. For that reason when human and nonhuman animals eat medicinal plants they are freed from Hunger and become active.

> Prajāpati consumed the most essential juice of those plants, and because of this he was completely satisfied. Human and nonhuman animals, however, eat the remaining juice [i.e., not the most nourishing juices] of the medicinal plants, and that is why earthly creatures get hungry from day to day.
>
> Prajāpati then placed Hunger in Time, whereupon Time became hungry. Time then began to feast on the gods and the demons, who, being eaten by Time, sought Prajāpati's protection. Prajāpati told them about the elixir of immortality. They churned [the cosmic ocean], and the elixir of immortality emerged [from it].[28]
>
> "But who would consume the elixir first?" Old Reviver asked Kaśyapa.
>
> The gods alone consumed it, and they became forever young and immortal. Because of the elixir of immortality, the gods thwarted Hunger and Time. Snubbed by the gods in this way, Time thus wears away all earthly creatures.
>
> The demons then converged on the gods, and the two groups fought. A young demoness named Long Tongue (Dīrghajihvī)[29] started destroying the army of the gods, who collectively called out to Skanda, their military leader: "Long Tongue is attacking us with great might. Control her!"
>
> "Choose a boon," Skanda replied.
>
> The gods said, "Oṃ."
>
> Skanda said, "Let me become one of the Vasus, one of the Rudras, and one of the Ādityas."[30]
>
> The gods again said, "Oṃ." And Skanda transformed.[31]

Kaśyapa then presents a lengthy list of the divine members of the Vasu, Rudra, and Āditya lineages to Old Reviver. He furthermore explains to Old Reviver that Skanda is known as the king of the three worlds, lord of the Vedic hymns, and commander of the gods. People who know this and properly venerate him, Kaśyapa asserts, succeed and enjoy wealth in their lives.[32] After this devotional excursus on the magnificence of Skanda, Kaśyapa narrates the events that led to the occurrence of miscarriage:

> Skanda then sent the goddess Revatī to fight Long Tongue. Revatī took the form of a she-jackal, approached the army of demons, and immediately devoured Long Tongue. After killing the young demoness, Revatī turned into a vulture.

> With meteors, lightning, and a rain of stones, Revatī, the Many-Formed One, raining all weapons, conquered the demons. Because they were being annihilated by the Many-Formed One, the demons absconded to the wombs of human and nonhuman animals. Revatī saw where the demons went, and immediately she became Jātahāriṇī, Seizer of the Born, and killed them.[33]

Character Sketches

Unlike the medical narrative of fever discussed in Chapter 3, which was based on a very old and well-known mythology, the "Destruction of Dakṣa's Sacrifice," before it was adapted to the *Carakasaṃhitā*, a number of the characters in the *Kāśyapasaṃhitā*'s miscarriage narrative are not as storied in Sanskrit literature. I thus offer a brief history of them here before embarking on my three-part analysis of the narrative.

In addition to her role in the Kaśyapa's compendium, several different characters named Revatī appear in Sanskrit literature. Her name is derived from the adjective *revat*, meaning "wealthy," "opulent," and "beautiful." In Hindu mythology, Revatī's most famous role is as the daughter of Raivata (also known as Kakudmin), king of the Ānarta province (modern-day western Gujarat), which is the region where Dvāraka, home of the god Kṛṣṇa, was located according to Hindu tradition. According to the *Bhāgavata Purāṇa*, Raivata was so enthralled by the beauty and giftedness of his daughter that he thought no mortal man was worthy of having her hand in marriage. He consulted the god Brahmā about future suitors for Revatī, and after ruminating on Raivata's concern for many eons, Brahmā decided that Balarāma, elder brother of Kṛṣṇa, should marry her.[34] Revatī and Balarāma married and eventually had two sons, Niṣṭha and Ulmuka. The name Revatī also regularly appears in Vedic astrology, where Revatī is the name of the fifth constellation;[35] in Varāhamihira's classic work on astronomy, the *Bṛhatsaṃhitā*, Revatī is the twenty-fifth constellation (*nakṣatra*).[36] Revatī is also the proper name of a series of chants in the *Chāndogya Upaniṣad*, the "Revatī Sāman chants woven upon animals," which brings good fortune, fame, and health to the person who knows and recites them.[37]

Especially germane to the present study are aspects of Revatī's mythological pedigree in the *Mahābhārata*, the *Suśrutasaṃhitā*, and the *Aṣṭāṅgahṛdayasaṃhitā*. In these three sources, Revatī is the name of one of the nine "child seizers" (*bālagrahas*) who take possession of (typically causing seizures) and cause health problems for small children.[38] Jean Filliozat's important study of the *Kumāra Tantra*, a Sanskrit treatise on pediatrics, lists twelve so-called Skanda-seizers, one of whom is called Śuṣkarevatī, "Emaciated Revatī." A child seized by Śuṣkarevatī suffers from fever, becomes emaciated, cries a great deal, and clinches his or her fists. As I discuss below, the *Kāśyapasaṃhitā* itself draws a direct connection between Revatī in the miscarriage narrative and the mythological line of child seizers in giving Revatī the epithet Pilipicchikā, which is the name of one of the twelve child seizers in the *Kumāra Tantra*.[39] David White has convincingly argued that the child seizers are linked to the Vedas, most notably the *Kauśika Sūtra* of the *Atharvaveda*, in which nine child seizers are collectively referred to as the names of the mothers (*mātṛnāmans*). The names of the mothers, White demonstrated, were intended to be used against attacks from Gandharvas, nymphs, demons, and other unwanted guests. Above all, the names of the mothers were to be sung as hymns to the female "seizers" (*grahīs*) in the course of sacrificial performance. The seizers of the *Atharvaveda* are the forerunners of classical medical and demonological figures like Revatī and Jātahāriṇī.[40]

Jātahāriṇī is not as common as Revatī in Sanskrit literature. In the Hindu mythological context, she is known as a menace to pregnant women and young children, much as she is in Kaśyapa's compendium. For instance, in the *Mārkaṇḍeya Purāṇa*, she is a flesh-eating demoness who wreaks havoc on women who deliver babies in polluted areas; she also steals embryos from wombs, and in some instances she snatches newly born babies and replaces them with her own demonic offspring.[41]

Determining a satisfactory translation for the name "Jātahāriṇī" is a challenging task. Dominik Wujastyk has translated her name as "Childsnatcher."[42] More often than not, scholars of Āyurveda and Indian medical history who mention Jātahāriṇi at all opt not to translate her name. P. V. Tewari, for instance, has written extensively on the *Kāśyapasaṃhitā* and the medical field of *kaumārabhṛtya*, and throughout her writings she lets Jātahāriṇī's story explain what her name denotes, rather than translating the name from the Sanskrit into English or Hindi.[43] Yet, because Sanskrit names often are very evocative of multiple layers of meaning, it can be helpful for our understanding of the stories in which they occur to translate them. Authors writing in Sanskrit in classical and medieval India regularly related a great deal about people and episodes in a story by ascribing certain names to people and places. In Hindu mythology, a name might encapsulate the general substance of a character. Take, for example, King Pāṇḍu in the *Mahābhārata*. His name means "Pale One" or "Impotent One." As his name suggests, he was unable to sire children. He was the father to the Pāṇḍava warriors, of course, but only because the gods, not he, impregnated his wives. Once we know the denotative substance of Pāṇḍu's name, we know a great deal about the narrative arc of his life—which is colored by ineffectualness and lack of vigor—and the heroic, divine-like feats of his sons in the epic. Conversely, a name might belie a character's qualities, such as in the case of Dakṣa, whom we saw in Chapter 3. The actions of Dakṣa, the "Able One" or "Intelligent One," in the *Carakasaṃhitā*'s medical narrative of fever reflect the antithesis of his sacrificial ability and acumen, thus underscoring the incongruity of his potential constructive behavior and the egregiousness of his actual behavior.

The name and character traits of Jātahāriṇī evoke Buddhist mythology and iconography. She is literally the "seizer" (*hāriṇī*) of things that have been "born" (*jāta*). Her actions in the miscarriage narrative have much in common with the Buddhist goddess Hārītī, who has been identified in sculptures at Gandhara during the Kuṣāṇa period (first to third centuries C.E.) and in the Buddhist cave temples at Ajanta (late fifth century C.E.).[44] The images of Hārītī that most closely resemble Jātahāriṇī, however, are found in Buddhist iconography in the cave temples of Ellora. Geri Malandra's masterful study of the temples at Ellora places the Elloran images of Hārītī around the seventh century C.E., which situates them at a time relatively coeval to the final redaction of the *Kāśyapasaṃhitā*. At Gandhara, Ajanta, and Ellora, Hārītī is generally depicted as the consort of Pāñcika, the leader of the *yakṣas*. Her story is instructive here for its historical and geographical markers, which are useful for making sense of the *Kāśyapasaṃhitā*'s depiction of the child-seizing Jātahāriṇī, who appears infrequently in Indian mythology, Hindu or otherwise. Associating Jātahāriṇī with the earliest images of Hārītī at Gandhara, circa the turn of the Common Era, suggests that the inspiration for the "Seizer of the Born" as a literary medical construct grew out of a wide-ranging geographic mixture of ideas among travelers, artisans, and traders on the routes of the Silk Road, where, around the second century B.C.E., Gandhara was a central stopover connecting Central Asia, northwestern India, and China. Furthermore, the connection of a narrative tradition in a Sanskrit medical source with long-standing Buddhist mythology is supported by the theory of Kenneth Zysk that the pioneers of classical Āyurveda lived among and shared their medical knowledge with itinerant, heterodox ascetic groups (*śramaṇas*) of Jains, Buddhists, and

Hindus in northwestern South Asia, dating back as early as the seventh century B.C.E.[45]

The stories of Hārītī and Jātahāriṇī are in fact quite similar. Hārītī undergoes a significant name change, from Abhiratī to Hārītī—that is, from "Pleasure" to "Seizer"—which marks the radical shift in her disposition and behavior. In Kaśyapa's compendium, Jātahāriṇī also undergoes a similar change, from Revatī to Jātahāriṇī—or from the "Opulent One" to "Seizer of the Born." Like Hārītī, during her metamorphosis, her disposition and modus operandi change considerably. Hārītī is a *yakṣa*, a frequently "anthropomorphized symbol of abundance, wealth, and fecundity" in Hinduism, echoing Jātahāriṇī's initial persona as Revatī.[46] The images of Hārītī at Ellora and Ajanta describe a legend about Hārītī from the *Lalitavistara*, a work from the early centuries of the Common Era recounting the legendary lives of the Buddha. In the legend, Hārītī and her husband, Pāñcika, had five hundred children. Hārītī quickly lost the necessary energy to feed them all, so for nourishment she decided to devour the children in the town of Rājagṛha. The Buddha reprimanded her for doing this by taking away Hārītī's youngest and most beloved daughter, Priyaṅkarā. This enraged Hārītī, and she vowed not to stop eating the children of Rājagṛha until she had Prinyaṅkarā back. In the end, the townsfolk of Rājagṛha calmed Hārītī down by promising to ensure that neither she nor her children would ever be without food.[47] David White has suggested that "Buddhist mythology tells us that Harītī's wrathful behavior stems from wrongs committed against her in a previous life: forced to dance at a festival while pregnant, she had miscarried and lost her child."[48] The conversion of Abhiratī from a pleasant mother and wife to the child-devouring, demonic figure of Hārītī parallels the *Kāśyapasaṃhitā*'s portrayal of Revatī, the insuperable defender of the godly cohort, into Jātahāriṇī, the terrifying Seizer of the Born.

In somatic and physiologic terms, the compendium of Kaśyapa identifies thirty-one classes of *jātahāriṇī*s—the medical condition, not the mythic demoness of the narrative. They have three modes of transmission: humans, animals, and divine beings.[49] Like most diseases in ayurvedic medicine, they have three prognoses: curable, treatable but not curable, and incurable.[50] Some *jātahāriṇī*s strike newborn children up to fifteen days after birth, whereas others clearly have an effect on embryos that are developing in the womb. The various *jātahāriṇī*s mentioned in the text are said to cause a range of different disorders, and each *jātahāriṇī* has a different name consistent with its target. Thus, *puṣpa jātahāriṇī* blocks the menstrual flow or causes an unproductive menstruation; *vikuṭā jātahāriṇī* causes irregular menstruation; *durdharā jātahāriṇī* causes fetal defects; *stambhanī jātahāriṇī* prevents the fetus from moving in utero; and so on. A major difference between the *jātahāriṇī* that seizes a newborn and the *jātahāriṇī* that seizes an embryo is that the former directly strikes the baby, whereas the latter affects the embryo by striking the pregnant woman.[51] The *jātahāriṇī* in the medical narrative of miscarriage above is specifically *the* Seizer of the Born. She is Jātahāriṇī with a capital *J*, of whom there are thirty-one subtypes. This story presents the important moment of the origination of miscarriage on earth. In doing so in an intricate narrative form, the authors of Kaśyapa's compendium assemble a biophysiologic etiology that may be interpreted using an array of hermeneutic approaches. Among the potential readings, in the remainder of this chapter I explore three somatic lessons that I regard as fundamental to the Revatī-Jātahāriṇī story. Although each reading differs slightly in its focus, insofar as I concentrate on the mythological components of the story or the question of authorship, each reading I offer has a pointed message pertaining to gender and the politics of gendered discourse

From Heaven to Earth, from Goddess to Avatar

As I have discussed elsewhere, Jātahāriṇī's act of eliminating demons from the wombs of human and nonhuman animals functions as an etiology for miscarriage in the *Kāśyapasaṃhitā*. The female womb is portrayed as the frontline in the din of battle between gods and demons over the right to immortality. The location of the womb is concurrently coincidental, serving as it did as a hiding place on earth for the demons fleeing from Jātahāriṇī, and highly significant, for on account of Jātahāriṇī's aggressive assault the production of offspring in the human and animal worlds seemingly lies in the balance.[52]

The etiological narrative of miscarriage in the *Kāśyapasaṃhitā* follows a standard pattern in Hindu mythology: a god(dess) is called upon to kill a demon(ess), but the demon(ess) flees and takes refuge in a human body. Following the demons that inhabit the wombs of female human and nonhuman animals, Revatī's avatar, Jātahāriṇī, travels to earth and possesses the very same bodies the demons possess. It is of course the nature of an avatar to move from the heavens to the human world. This is the literal "descent" (*avatāra*) of deities that enables the interface of gods and humans in Sanskrit literature and Hindu mythology. The most well known *avatāras* in Hinduism are the ten descents, or earthly incarnations, of the god

Viṣṇu, two of which have been for centuries enormously popular and religiously significant Hindu deities in their own right: Rāma and Kṛṣṇa. The goddess Revatī and her *avatāra*, Jātahāriṇī, share a typical trans-world relationship, which in the miscarriage narrative allows them to intersect and inhabit both the divine and human worlds. Their association also presents us, the readers, with two distinctive angles from which to make sense of the picture of miscarriage that is recounted in this medical text. From a cosmological perspective, for example, Jātahāriṇī's demon-slaying occupation may be read as an important recalibration of the relationship between the earthly and heavenly realms within the universal order. That is, it is the primeval nature of the demonic cohort in Indian mythology to dwell alongside and opposed to the gods in the heavenly realm, not hiding in the wombs of human women and female animals. The removal of the demons from their unnatural dwelling restores the cosmological balance of existence for the residents of the heavens and earth. Read in this way Jātahāriṇī acts like a divine physician, restoring order to a cosmic physiology that had gone askew. The forcible elimination of the demons, who, after occupying the wombs of earthly females, the compendium's authors later recast in the role as gestating embryos or fetuses, is fundamental to the task of supporting the proper functioning of the universe. Viewed from a more local, telluric perspective, the avataric conversion of Revatī into Jātahāriṇī may be read as an indispensable act for the prevention of the proliferation of demons on earth. This reading indicates there might be an advantage to Jātahāriṇī's hostile treatment of a woman's womb—namely, that Jātahāriṇī decisively eliminates the danger of a woman carrying to term and giving birth to a demon-child. Such a perspective is, to be sure, problematic given the physical trouble and emotional suffering that often accompany miscarriage. Yet it is a viable reading, and we need to query the narrative and the broader context of the *Kāśyapasaṃhitā* as to why this type of narrative logic might have been used in the coverage of miscarriage.

In what we have seen thus far of the miscarriage narrative, the annexation of a woman's womb by a demon appears to be arbitrary. The text does not suggest, in other words, that a demon takes possession of a womb owing to a fault of the woman. The ostensibly neutral position that women are unsuspecting victims swiftly changes, however. The biophysical event of miscarriage is woven together with socioreligious agency and especially Hindu dharma, as we see in the following passage listing the reasons why Jātahāriṇī enters certain women.

> Jātahāriṇī kills the menstrual flow. She kills the body. She kills the embryos; she kills [children] that have been born; she kills [fetuses] being born; and she kills [embryos] that will be born. She principally kills the demonic offspring of people without dharma and those infected with non-dharma. Old Reviver, that is her, Revatī! She is the Many-Formed One, Seizer of the Born, also known as Pilipicchikā.[53] She is said to be a descendent of Rudra and a descendant of Varuṇa. She is the one who, at Skanda's command, has come into being among all creatures to remove untruths and stupefy those who act against dharma.
>
> O' Old Reviver, now we will explain the primary cause of Revatī, her emergence, and her symptoms, how to get rid of her, and the medicine to alleviate her.
>
> Old Reviver asks: "Why is it that good people, too, are killed when the evil demons get inside them?"
>
> That is because when Jātahāriṇī gets inside them, only someone with a divine eye can see that she is there [inside an apparently good person, and therefore it appears that a good person is being killed]. And so it is said that only by following dharma can a woman stop Jātahāriṇī [from getting inside her].[54]

A lucid, authorial voice intimating a set of anxieties about the bodies of women and their social behaviors comes through here in the character of Kaśyapa, who declares to Old Reviver that Revatī's motivations for generating miscarriage in the human world are in fact pointedly marked at certain women. Next, the compilers of the *Kāśyapasaṃhitā* cast Revatī's avatar, Jātahāriṇī, as an assessor of right and wrong behavior, for she is said, again through the character mouthpiece of the medical sage Kaśyapa, to alight only on women who are morally errant.

> Jātahāriṇī attaches to any woman who has abandoned dharma, auspicious behavior, cleanliness, and sacrifice to the gods; she attaches to any woman who hates gods, cows, brahmins, teachers, elders, and good people; she attaches to any woman who is fickle, egoistic, and dissolute; she attaches to any woman who loves hostility, discord, meat, violence, sleep, and sex; she attaches to any woman who is cruel, causes torment, is caustic, chatty, or unjust . . .[55]

Jātahāriṇī also afflicts women who do not submit to the will of their husbands or love their children; who despise their in-laws; give their co-wives the evil eye; hit babies on the head; and fail to sacrifice to the ancestors. The list is extensive. Because of one or a combination of these misdeeds, a woman creates openings in her body (literally "doors," *dvāreṣu*) through which Jātahāriṇī may enter and then attach to her womb.

In the course of the narrative, it becomes clear the compilers of Kaśyapa's compendium wanted to establish culpability for the occurrence of miscarriage, which now appears to be a kind of punishment for a woman's depravity, immorality, and general misconduct. The narration turns miscarriage into the secondary theme of the story, in fact, shifting the focus onto the actions of women, and portraying miscarriage as a medical outcome of social and ethical activity. What's more, the biophysical misfortune of miscarriage, illustrated in the story as Jātahāriṇī effectively cleansing a woman's womb in response to the woman's misdeeds, is not just a somatic lesson for women who are currently pregnant. The lesson is for women of childbearing age across the board. It is for any woman who can become pregnant. The demons that escaped to the wombs of women in the opening segment of the narrative are metaphors for the latent socioreligious deviancy that morally errant women could reproduce among the human population. It is always important to remember, as I discuss below, this heavy-handed ethical exposé of women is the product of male authors, who ultimately chose what is socially and religiously acceptable for women. For these authors the Jātahāriṇī character is the key part to piece together a cultural puzzle that presents the reproductive and gynecologic well-being of a woman as the result of, not to mention coterminous with, an exhaustive normative code of duties and proscriptions. This code is one of the many variants of what I have called elsewhere, and what I discuss at length in Chapter 7, the unique "body dharma" of Āyurveda, cast here in a highly gender-specific mold.[56]

As the narrative changes from the mythical etiology of miscarriage to a palpable declaration about a human woman's body dharma, which is to say, the somatic bases of a woman's interpersonal obligations and ritual expectations in Hindu society, the authors of Kaśyapa's compendium actively ethicize. Storytelling is their medium to invest ethical elements into their medical discourse, and the patient is the prototype upon which they illustrate their normative agenda. To read narrative medical discourse in classical Āyurveda with the intention of understanding its meaning and consequence for classical Indian society (and later Indian societies, too, where the literature continues to be influential), we must treat the literature as the product of a culturally embedded knowledge system, which was produced by authors who envisioned "long life" (*āyus*) and health of the body to be contingent upon the diverse domains, actors, and institutions in society. Ayurvedic chart talk in the Sanskrit classics is denuded of claims to authority on anything other than knowledge of the workings of the human body. Contrastingly, the narrative literature involves the presentation of situations leading to ill health and somatic malfunction, which openly suggest that the people who depict these situations and unhealthy and somatically faulty people (the medical patients, or rogins) assert a kind of social and/or religious authority. Narrative medical discourse in these cases reveals a high level of religious ideology and moralizing in the construction of the ayurvedic patient. In this regard, the Indian literary context presents a very different perspective than what has been studied in recent scholarship in narrative medical ethics in the United States, where physicians, anthropologists, and sociologists have documented stories of illness reported by medical patients. In India, in the literature of Āyurveda, we do not have documentation of the patient's perspective. Eminent scholars studying biomedicine from social science and humanities perspectives, such as Arthur Kleinman, Rita Charon, Cheryl Mattingly, Susan Sontag, and others, have illuminated the study of the doctor–patient exchange in Western biomedicine by giving voice to, and elucidating the importance of, the travails and experiences of the individuals who receive biomedical treatment. These people—the patients—are often overlooked in discussions of technological prowess and advancements in biomedical research. Yet, opportunities for patients to share their illness narratives and the trials of coming to terms with the condition of patienthood have proven to be therapeutic. These stories have also functioned as a kind of ethical audit of biomedical education and the ways in which physicians are trained for clinical practice and research. The voices and experiences of patients of classical Āyurveda are not exactly present in the Sanskrit medical literature. They must be inferred, as I explain in Chapter 7, and pieced together on the basis of the medical authors' presentations of pathology and disease. To explain illness, somatic malfunction, and patienthood, the authors of the Sanskrit medical classics sometimes adumbrate ethical imperatives for people to follow. This happens most clearly in the construction of narrative medicine. Narrativizing in the medical context Hindu myths and weighty religious concepts like dharma and karma, the compilers of classical ayurvedic literature projected a medical agenda that both actively contributed to discussions about the make up of human culture and generated codes of conduct for the day-to-day negotiation of social relationships and institutions that constitute human life.

So we return to the medical stories, to the literary presentation of wellness and illness, and we are confronted with very involved turns of phrase, character sketches, and intratextual allusions, all of which contribute to our understanding of patienthood in the classical medical sources. In the miscarriage narrative, Revatī's avatar is among the most evocative literary elements. The authorial change in tone and focus in the story from mythic etiology to ethical fiat mirrors the change in Revatī from battler of the demons to Jātahāriṇī, Seizer of the Born and handler of procreational affairs on earth. This shift in focus, I suggest, invites an interpretation of "Jātahāriṇī" as a metonym for miscarriage in a dual sense—in the physiologic sense as the sudden expulsion of an embryo from the womb and in the socioethical sense of a failure to bring about some desired end. The Jātahāriṇī character equally represents the embodiment of embryonic ruin and a woman's socioreligious failure to act according to a certain code of conduct. As in the preceding passages of the miscarriage story, dharma—in this case a violation of dharma—is the baseline the text's evaluation of women. In the narrative terms the *Kāśyapasaṃhitā* establishes, dharma is the central motivating factor in Jātahāriṇī's attack:

> Jātahāriṇī does not enter the womb of the woman who obeys dharma. She is driven by the absence of dharma against the mother, father, and sons. . . . whereupon [she causes] the destruction of the offspring of mothers. Because of [a woman's] own actions, Jātahāriṇī makes the lives of children come to an end.[57]

The *Kāśyapasaṃhitā* only provides details about the women in whom Jātahāriṇī settles, not the women whom she disregards. The women on whom she alights appear to possess perceived character traits that stand opposed to more presumably upright and honorable temperaments, temperaments that do not invite a visit from Jātahāriṇī. Lists of social and physical attributes that define the feminine nature, or a woman's disposition in relation to others, are not uncommon in Āyurveda.[58] Often, though not always, in the narrative discourses of the Sanskrit medical literature, as we see here in the compendium of Kaśyapa, positive feminine qualities are discernable via negativa. As readers, we may indirectly determine the qualities and actions of women that are not likely to invite Jātahāriṇī into their lives. Hence, a woman to whom Jātahāriṇī would pay no attention might be socially and religiously virtuous, dharmically vigilant, altruistic, agreeable, sexually modest, and the like.

The fundamental somatic lesson of this medical narrative, the veritable moral of the story, is that miscarriages occur because of social and religious failings. The medical narrative in this case is a heuristic device that the authors of the *Kāśyapasaṃhitā* used to appropriate and rationalize certain religious concepts and ideas into their medical program, most notably dharma but also the relationship between gods and humans. Maneuvering a plurality of codes, the medical authors make use of language to form a highly polysemous text that systematically arranges rules and regulations apropos cultural and religious norms that permeate the setting and characters of the story.[59] The narrative time and rationale of the story involve a process of linking a set of relations—gods and demons—to an otherwise unrelated situation—human miscarriage—in order to address issues the text's authors wanted to underscore. For this literary undertaking to work, the narrative must progress seamlessly across its various codes of meaning. Gods and demons and women and miscarriage all must fit together in such a way that shifting settings and temporal frames in the narrative—heavenly space and time and earthly space and time—appear to exist in a fluid course of association. Accordingly, the *Kāśyapasaṃhitā*'s story renders the character and conduct of women comprehensible by way of comparison to the heavenly realm. The paired character of Revatī-Jātahāriṇī enables this translation of one realm into another, that is, from the heavenly into the human. While Revatī upholds cosmic order by reorganizing the divine contradistinction of gods and demons in the heavens, Jātahāriṇī cultivates the social order on earth by mediating and controlling what goes on in the lives and wombs of women.

In Chapter 1, I suggested that a vital function of the medical narrative is to press an "ought" into service among a community of people, in effect to move from a theoretical ethic to an applied ethic via medical discourse that uses a sociological idiom. This begs the question: what evidence do we have that the *Kāśyapasaṃhitā* (or the medical literature of the period in general) was applied and its information disseminated? Moreover, for whom was the narrative knowledge specifically designed? As is the case with the other ayurvedic classics, such as the *Carakasaṃhitā* and *Suśrutasaṃhitā*, the *Kāśyapasaṃhitā* is organized as a manual and it was, as best as we can determine, composed primarily for and by vaidyas. In the particular case of Kaśyapa's compendium, the principal original audience would therefore have been physicians trained specifically in the fields of pediatrics, obstetrics, and embryology (*kaumārabhṛtya*). The classical Sanskrit medical sources were not simply static archival products, however. They were composed for use. And they were composed of knowledge that was meant to be disseminated in one way or another. Apart from physicians trained in *kaumārabhṛtya*, we know that the audience of the physicians who used Kaśyapa's compendium would have been primarily women, but also possibly children. Yet the ways in which, as well as the extent to which, classical Indian physicians made the technical material in their texts available to their patients is difficult to know with absolute certainty. That the medical narratives of ayurvedic literature, which contrast sharply with the chart talk of the literature, are filled with popular cultural stories and concepts suggests that they might have had been intended for an audience larger than just the professional medical community. Fundamentally, establishing a favorable reception of the character and idea of Jātahāriṇī among both medical professionals and patients is ultimately an effort to take control of, and hence look after, human reproduction. An obvious reason for this is that procreation has been an enormously important issue in the history of South Asia, and within the history of Hinduism in particular. For example, important Hindu resources on dharma, most notably *The Laws of Manu*, eulogize women as goddesses for their power to generate human life.[60] Perhaps more significant to the case at hand, in several Brāhmaṇas and the *Mahābhārata*, embryological matters and reproduction appear to be as vital, if not demonstrably more vital, to men as they are to women. In these sources, men are said to be "debtors" (*ṛṇavans*) at birth by virtue of their gender. In the Brāhmaṇas, a man is born with three debts (*ṛṇas*): a debt of Vedic study to the rishis, a debt of sacrifice to the gods, and a debt of offspring to the ancestors;[61] in the *Mahābhārata*, an additional fourth debt of benevolence to all mankind is added.[62] To be free of the debt to the ancestors, which is the debt most clearly endangered in the *Kāśyapasaṃhitā*'s miscarriage narrative, a man needed to have offspring, preferably sons, to perform his funeral rites (*śrāddha*) and ensure his immortality after death.[63]

The Jātahāriṇī character brings to pass the sociological objective of the text's authors: to control human procreation in order to establish an enduring patriline of descent. And yet it is noteworthy that, for all of this medical narrative's androcentric aims and foci, the *Kāśyapasaṃhitā* does not let men completely off the hook for a woman's miscarriage. Men bear some of the responsibility for a visitation from Jātahāriṇī. If a husband's activities cascade into egoism, sexual recklessness, and the like, he too may bid Jātahāriṇī's descent.

A man may catch Jātahāriṇī (in the sense that we typically say someone "catches" a cold) after having contact with a woman who has already been seized by Revatī's avatar. That is, a man commonly catches Jātahāriṇī after committing adultery. He will, unless he performs special atonement rituals, undoubtedly pass Jātahāriṇī on to his wife the next time he "goes to her."[64] This means that men and husbands may carry Jātahāriṇī, too; however, they endure no physical harm themselves from the experience. Instead, men are social vectors for Jātahāriṇī, passing her along from one woman to another. In this way, men function as links in a chain of transmission via human-to-human contact, and thereby facilitate Jātahāriṇī's seizures of women.[65] Despite the absence of physical affliction, men do suffer a potentially great loss when Jātahāriṇī induces miscarriage in their spouses. They lose the opportunity to have sons, and therefore run the risk of remaining scofflaws on their debts to the ancestors in the present life, through their transmigratory journey, and into their next lifetimes.

Reality and Experience: Men Attending to Women's Bodies

Like all of the Sanskrit medical classics, the *Kāśyapasaṃhitā* was composed and compiled by men. As a result, the text presents ideas and depicts visions of medical etiologies through the eyes of men. The authorial voice in the foregoing narrative about miscarriage is contained in the Revatī–Jātahāriṇī character. She controls what the male authors would like to control. As Wendy Doniger and Sudhir Kakar have noted of "male texts" in ancient India, in general the male composers "merely engage in a ventriloquism that attributes to women viewpoints that in fact serve male goals."[66] The gods and goddesses of the *Kāśyapasaṃhitā*'s narrative of failed pregnancies are abstract projections of empirical aspirations of the human authors of the narrative. Put another way, the divine beings in the story serve as "supernatural standard-bearers," who, following Brian Smith's reading of divinities in Indian myths, represent particular qualities people in society ought to possess and mimic.[67] The narrativization of miscarriage in the *Kāśyapasaṃhitā* demonstrates that the field of medicine in classical India occupied, and indeed actively sought to occupy, sociocultural spaces in which the body is seen not simply as an anatomical unit. The placement of narrative discourse in the medical domain encourages an expansive view of the body by both physician and patient as an instrument with which people directly experience the world of objects and thereafter bring their individual lives to bear on other people and various aspects of society, such as the structure of domestic life and family hierarchies, gender relations, and religious practice.

Men mediate and ultimately control the depiction of women that reaches the audience of the narrative origins of miscarriage in the compendium of Kaśyapa. The handling of the goddess Revatī in the narrative illustrates this point well. She is a strong goddess, and she accomplishes a great task that the entire legion of gods could not perform. She single-handedly destroys Long Tongue (Dīrghajihvī) and countless other demons. But at the end of the day, the power of Revatī manifests only when the chief god, Skanda, authorizes her to act. She has the means to defeat many foes only if her male superior commands her to do so. The events depicting the gods' struggle for, and eventual attainment of, the nectar of immortality in heaven are analogous to the desire on the part of the authors of the miscarriage narrative to control the activities of pregnant women and to ensure the safe production of healthy male children on earth. The demons' retreat to the wombs of human and nonhuman animals suggests that those tasked with the arrangement and dissemination of the medical knowledge of the *Kāśyapasaṃhitā* perceived the womb to be not only a highly important biological sanctuary for the production of children, especially male children, but it was also an organ in the female body that was prone to pestiferous and potentially fatal corruption. It therefore occupied a great deal of attention in classical ayurvedic literature, nowhere more so than among medical specialists of *kaumārabhṛtya*.

The *Kāśyapasaṃhitā*'s authors attempted to mitigate the potential corruption of the womb by listing punishable, or miscarriage-inducing, activities women should avoid. For example, the text enjoins first-time pregnant women to avoid the sight of wicked people, literally any people who might be "bad-selved" (*durātman*), a term that conjures a profoundly venal type of personality given the generally incorruptible nature of the self (or ātman) in Hinduism. Earlier we saw that Jātahāriṇī attacks the badly behaved woman who actively casts an evil eye at one of her co-wives. A. Stewart Woodburne has written about the folkloric traditions of the evil eye, called *dṛṣṭi*, "sight." Women, he explains, are regularly portrayed casting the evil eye out of feelings of jealousy and spite. In Hinduism, the evil eye is also commonly associated with pregnancy and birth, as Woodburne explains:

> The Hindu belief is that the crises of life are particularly precarious from the standpoint of susceptibility to the evil eye. So at times of childbirth, puberty and marriage one

> must be more than usually careful to take precautions against evil influences. . . . Much care must be taken as to the objects that a woman sees during pregnancy, as it will affect her child.[68]

In the Hindu context, references to the power of sight immediately call to mind religious "viewing," *darśana*, (or in Hindi, *darśan*, without the final *'a,'* as it is frequently heard across north India), in which a devotee and a deity unite through visual contact. But rather than an auspicious viewing in which a devotee momentarily unites with the divine, through sight, as in darśan, the consequences of the pregnant woman's ill-projected sight—the evil eye—and the sighting of a pregnant woman by people with bad selves ultimately invite Jātahāriṇī to destroy a developing embryo. Oddly, the situation of the pregnant woman corresponds to the deity's image in the religious act of darśan insofar as she is perceived to have provocatively presented herself, as the deity presents itself, for public viewing. Nevertheless, the *Kāśyapasaṃhitā* is clear that the pregnant woman does not receive Jātahāriṇī as a result of presenting herself for an endearing spouse or relative, but rather for people with bad selves:

> When a woman is pregnant for the first time, she is free of disease, she has a beautiful body, round buttocks, milk-filled breasts . . . she has good hair . . . [and] an increasing linea negra, resplendent hands, feet, nails, eyes, and skin. She is intelligent and delicate. At this time, if people with bad selves see the pregnant woman, and if she does not perform the pacification rituals, Jātahāriṇī will prey on her. For that reason, it is said that the woman desirous of sons should everyday perform a sacrifice for what is desired.[69]

The male authors of this text also describe the somatic characteristics common in women seized by Jātahāriṇī: the woman's body withers; she becomes anxious and malnourished; her mind becomes unsteady and her immunity breaks down; she loses her livestock, her reputation is defamed, and she becomes a widow.[70]

On the whole, the medical narratives of Āyurveda conform to the overall aim of the medical system, which is to ensure long life among patients through the distribution of knowledge about how to achieve and maintain health. The story of Revatī–Jātahāriṇī was meant to educate women about pregnancy and thereby ensure safe pregnancies. But there is more. Medical stories about the human body like the

Kāśyapasaṃhitā's miscarriage narrative introduce causes of ill health that implicate the social and religious communities of patients. There is a lot to be won or lost in the event of a miscarriage. As we have seen, men stand to lose a great deal in their afterlives if they do not successfully produce sons. Medical storytelling turns out to be more than just a means for biological discussion, because the socioreligious implications of miscarriage for men appear to be as important as, if not more important than, the physical ramifications women might suffer from enduring a miscarriage. This is a distinctly gendered somatic lesson, and it outlines a classic hierarchical relationship between men and women on earth by analogy with the pecking order of the gods and demons in the heavens. After the demons fail in their battle against the gods for immortality, they take refuge in the wombs of women. The backdrop of the heavens, set in the timelessness of mythic imagery, and the perennial tussle between the gods and demons for immortality serves as a prelude to the narrative relocation in the world of humans, where the primary concern is the Hindu religious aim to establish a solid patriline that will ensure safe passage for male elders in saṃsāra. Myth effectively becomes medical commentary on the social and religious lives of women. In particular, the text envisions women's physicality during pregnancy and the childbearing years as highly tenuous. Female fragility at these times is furthermore said to be intensified, indeed prone to slide into biological malfunction, including miscarriage, by an apparent propensity to be involved, whether directly or indirectly, in questionable behavior.

The gender dyad at work in the miscarriage narrative at first appears rather straightforward. It is common to find in the Sanskrit medical classics, as well as other Sanskrit literatures from classical and medieval India, men producing texts that constructively ethicize social and religious roles for women with an endgame that fixes advantages for the male authors over against the female objects of study. Nonetheless, for modern readers of the miscarriage myth in the *Kāśyapasaṃhitā* it is somewhat puzzling to encounter what appears to be detailed knowledge about the somatic experience of embryonic ruin, miscarriage, when it is a physical experience the authors of the text would never have had. Of course, medical authors write about diseases and bodily dysfunctions they may never have or experience directly. I am not suggesting that men cannot or should not comment on, or become specialists in, embryology or obstetrics. What I am suggesting is that the function of this medical narrative is not to describe the embodied reality of miscarriage. The narrative reverses the way in which an audience would "read" the somatic experience of miscarriage.

Instead of presenting miscarriage as a crisis originating in the body and then laying out the ramifications of that crisis on the pregnant woman and those around her, the story starts with the effects and then moves backwards to the cause. It presents a socioethical paper trail of misdeeds and misconduct—to wit, social miscarriages—one after the other, establishing a line of events causatively leading to a woman's womb and the termination of her pregnancy. The story line that follows Revatī's transformation into Jātahāriṇī offers the rationalization that embryonic ruin is the natural outcome of certain violations of religious knowledge and social behaviors.

Refraining from the largely unbiased biological discourse characteristic of ayurvedic chart talk, the *Kāśyapasaṃhitā*'s account of miscarriage is a narrative of moral normativity. A woman's embodied perception actually posits the reality of miscarriage, and the authors attempt to deal with this issue by reflecting, or illuminating, the medical reality perceptible to them, which is a reality they can never experience or know firsthand. The narrative is an exercise in the phenomenology of already constituted cultural categories, such as men and women, gods and demons, creation, human life, and social duty. Female subjecthood during pregnancy is bankrupt in the story. It has to be that way. All life events touch and provoke people's relationships, behaviors, and tastes in ways that are truly known only to the people perceiving them. At best, the men who prepared this story could identify women's tastes, attitudes, and characters as they relate to this medical matter through a study of the social context in which women live. Kenneth Zysk has shown that this line of thinking, in which a "fundamental association existed between the ailment and its perceived cause," occurs very early in the history of medicine in India.[71] Yet the logic typically follows a pattern in which internal, invisible ailments are understood to derive from unseen causes, such as gods and demons, and external or visible suffering is attributable to seen causes, such as blunt trauma from physical objects. Conversely, the story of miscarriage in the *Kāśyapasaṃhitā* attempts to link what is portrayed as an unseen, internal affliction—miscarriage, also known as Jātahāriṇī—with a visible, external cause—the social behaviors of women. The narrative and its subsequent rationalization thus express men's observations and preconceived notions about the company women prefer to keep and the places where they prefer to be.

The experiences of other people can be recorded, tallied, and assessed. They cannot be replicated. Because women have a special knowledge of their bodies and an inherent somatic means of attention concerning procreation that men do not have we might ask: how could the authors of Kaśyapa's compendium, all of whom were surely male, squarely or thoroughly treat these experiences of the body? The fact is they could neither properly start nor end their analysis at the basic level of being and experience, which is intimately tied to perception. Perception in Āyurveda stands solely in the body, with the sense organs (*indriyas*), which I discussed in Chapter 2. For that reason, this medical narrative starts where perception and experience end. It starts with the objects and results of embodied living in the world. Adapted to the medical compendium of Kaśyapa from Hindu and Buddhist mythology, the Revatī-Jātahāriṇī narrative presents a rationalization for the social and ethical causes of miscarriage first and foremost, not the biophysical sources or consequences of the event. The nature of the medical narrative in Āyurveda is to present easily identifiable somatic lessons, instructions about how to use the body in one's daily engagements with other people, as an instrument of religious practice and, as we find in the origin story of miscarriage discussed here, as a vital mechanism in the construction and preservation of family and society. With these objectives, the tale of Revatī-Jātahāriṇī and the origins of miscarriage are meant to influence the hearts and minds of the *Kāśyapasaṃhitā*'s audience. The *Kāśyapasaṃhitā* is of course a medical treatise, a textbook referred to and referenced primarily by specialists, and in general the audience of this text is circumscribed. But the narratives of the Sanskrit medical literature present us with something remarkably different from the chart talk of the tradition, which is clearly designed for a limited group of people—practicing vaidyas and medical educators—for whom content such as the minutiæ of biological indexes, nosological taxonomies, botanical preparations, and the like would be intelligible and therefore meaningful. The medical narratives offer up a different kind of literature, the medical usage and audience of which is far less limited. The aims of these stories appear to be about the persuasion and nurturance of the minds of an audience, which in the case of the miscarriage narrative in particular includes women who are pregnant and of childbearing age and the male vaidyas who counsel and treat them. In the *Kāśyapasaṃhitā*, the Revatī-Jātahāriṇī account of why a woman might have experienced a miscarriage or what could befall a women when she becomes pregnant is designed to encourage people to rethink their positions on the ideas of women's subjecthood and agency using the morally-laden lens of the medical narrative's presentation of reality.[72]

A feminine perspective on the experience of miscarrying a fetus is absent from the account of miscarriage in the *Kāśyapasaṃhitā*. The text does not indicate that women were in conversation with this source's compilers. A female perspective is rare in Sanskrit literature by and large, but it is not unheard of in the medical context. Martha Ann Selby has written about a group of "accomplished women" (*āptā striyaḥ*) in an extended birth narrative in the *Carakasaṃhitā*, who appear as a chorus of elder and knowledgeable women in the delivery room of a primipara. These women offer guidance and relate information to the younger, expectant mother, always at the command of the physician.[73] The compilers of the *Carakasaṃhitā* communicate precious little information about whom these accomplished women might have been, apart from describing their activities during delivery. It is thus difficult to know the extent to which they actually contributed to or influenced the data about delivery presented in the work. The women are said to have been "sympathetic" (*anukūlā*), however, and they are said to have sung hymns of joy as the primipara worked to bring forth her baby. This suggests that these women did contribute, at the very least, a sense of understanding and comfort to the environment of the classical ayurvedic delivery room.[74] Citing subtle turns of phrase in the text's discourse to describe the feeling and experience of giving birth, Selby reads a number of the comments of the *Carakasaṃhitā*'s male authors as patently more male than female in nature; there are other passages in the work, however, that she reads as clearly more female than male. Because of this, she reasons that there must have been an exchange of knowledge between women and men on matters of labor and delivery. Only women, for example, could describe the special pains of fetal loosening as "a feeling as if a bandage has been removed from the chest."[75] This and other examples leads Selby to conclude:

> In the *Āyurvedic* gynecological scenario, male empirical observation appears to fuse with female narratives, which results in extremely interesting and complex problems of gendered discourse; of male and female ways of knowing the female body according to its public and private, or rather, visible and invisible surfaces. I would hazard to say that in this particular instance, the usual entrenched gender hierarchies that we find inside these texts and out become confounded. Lines are blurred and erased in the creation of a ritual and medical technology that is driven by the urge to produce *śreyasī prajā*, the very best offspring.[76]

Unlike the *Carakasaṃhitā*, however, the *Kāśyapasaṃhitā* does not present us with similarly clear indicators that women were in any way involved in the adaptation of the Revatī–Jātahāriṇī narrative to the medical context.

The lines of a gendered hierarchy are not blurred in this medical narrative, as Selby found them to be in the birthing accounts in the *Carakasaṃhitā*. In fact, the very use of the Revatī–Jātahāriṇī story demonstrates an attempt by the compilers of the *Kāśyapasaṃhitā* to buttress the male way of knowing over against the female way of knowing on the matter of embryonic ruin, miscarriage, and its socio-religious associations. In the Revatī–Jātahāriṇī story, the entirety of the woman, her body and being in the world, becomes a vessel in which to produce and gestate an embryo, and eventually give birth to a baby. The woman literally becomes the womb. She is totally organic, a breathing machine, in the sense that her uterus subtends her whole nature. As a machine, when she acts, she runs the risk of breaking down. Machines are also manipulable. The presentation of miscarriage in Kaśyapa's compendium, in the Revatī-Jātahāriṇī story itself and the subsequent elaboration of what a "jātahāriṇī" is and does, serves up somatic lessons in this specific medical context that exploit this perceived manipulability.

Using the Revatī–Jātahāriṇī story, the *Kāśyapasaṃhitā*'s compilers effectively wrest control of women and human development from conception through gestation by co-opting women's power to define their somatic experiences for themselves. The story not only rewrites the female patient's somatic experience of miscarriage, but it also recounts that experience as an episode in a larger morality play about good and evil. This morality play is but a part of the grand narrative of "support for the young" (*kaumārabhṛtya*) in the entire work, which itself is an arm of the knowledge for long life (*āyurveda*) that defines the contours of classical Indian medicine. All of this knowledge surely does not come in the form of narrative discourse only. Where medical stories about the body serve as the platforms from which to impart medical knowledge, the ayurvedic compilers could secure the active consent of their patients to adopt not just their medical injunctions, but also the cultural values couched in their narratives. The adaptation of moral knowledge to the medical system in stories about the body facilitates a reformulation of common understandings of health and illness usually disseminated through standard chart talk, so that patients might begin to reexamine their illnesses along the normative lines of the narratives.

Nature versus Nurture

To conclude this chapter, I would like to consider briefly the story of miscarriage in Kaśyapa's compendium in light of a few age-old philosophical/medical/sociological questions about life, and in particular the question of nature versus nurture. Does nature (one's biology) or nurture (one's ecology) contribute more to the growth of a human being? To what degree are people born with the dispositions, tastes, and predilections they exhibit and act upon later in life? Are human beings hardwired at conception to act in certain ways throughout their lives, or do children and young adults develop inclinations and attitudes as they grow up amid family, make friends and foes, amass experiences, and undertake formal education?

There are proponents and detractors today on both sides of the nature–nurture debate. Most people, in the past as well as today, acknowledge that both biology and ecology influence who people are and what they become. Even before nature takes effect on the genetic material that becomes a new life, humans around the globe today, and equally so in ancient India, have come up with ways to try to fix the type of children they might have, as arranged marriages, in vitro fertilizations, consultations with astrologers and soothsayers, and the performance of certain sexual positions demonstrate. Yet it would seem that for the nine months following embryogenesis, pregnant women enjoy supreme control over the embryos developing in their wombs. The authors of the Revatī–Jātahāriṇī narrative address precisely this time and place, gestation and the womb, and argue that successful pregnancies are as contingent on the social relations of pregnant women as they are on women's personal biological cultivation.

The activities, diet, and mind-set of pregnant women can certainly have a great deal of influence on embryos in utero. In the classical Sanskrit medical literature of India, there is also a fair amount of discussion about the ways in which the embryo influences a pregnant woman. At a certain stage in pregnancy, for instance, the *Carakasaṃhitā* explains that "the embryo quickens and longs for whatever things he experienced in former lives. This is what old people call double-heartedness."[77] Double-heartedness (*dvaihṛdayya*) is said to occur at different times in the various compendia of Āyurveda but it typically occurs between the third and fourth months of pregnancy.[78] When it happens, the pregnant woman possesses two hearts, her own and the heart of her embryo. The line of influence between the pregnant woman and her embryo implied by the dual heart could hardly be more intimate. Pregnancy cravings and aversions are said to be the longings and dislikes of the growing embryo externalized through the pregnant woman's actions and tastes.[79] The double-hearted pregnant woman, furthermore, "should be given whatever she desires, except those things that cause damage to the embryo."[80] Pregnancy cravings, in other words, stem from the developing embryo as it wrestles with the memories, tastes, and cravings of its past lives. The wishes should be heeded and placated with due care because personal cultivation in this case, that is, a woman's hyper-refinement of her body through a heart-healthy diet and behavior, ensures an auspicious birth for the emerging fetus.

The medical source ascribed to Kaśyapa that I have been analyzing in this chapter does not discuss double-heartedness, but it clearly holds the position that things that are good for a pregnant woman also will be auspicious for her fetus. Such things include nutritional recommendations like a milk- and meat-based diets and certain social conventions to follow, including never wearing articles of clothing bearing feminine or gender-neutral imagery (which presumably would bring unwanted and potentially harmful attention to the pregnant woman from the wrong, or so-called bad-selved people).[81] The position of the *Kāśyapasaṃhitā* is not unlike biomedical discourse today, of which perhaps the most prominent and least-disputed argument is that pregnant women who smoke cigarettes, drink alcohol, and use drugs harm and possibly will destroy their embryos. Choices made and the company one keeps (nurture) are significant during the gestational period, even to the point of altogether overriding biology (nature). The modern campaign to discourage women from partaking of harmful substances during pregnancy has been, and continues to be, so pervasive, and comes from all corners of society (medicine, religion, politics, education, the media, and elsewhere), that few people today can honestly claim ignorance on this issue. The campaign has clear medical merit. But to put into service its evident value, the campaign must argue for and ultimately convince pregnant women to curtail certain social activities and make certain ethical choices.

The *Kāśyapasaṃhitā*'s miscarriage narrative demonstrates a combined religious (Hindu) and medical (Āyurveda) campaign from classical India that was designed to bring nurture into balance with nature in order to benefit embryological understanding and development. If there is medical merit to the argument in the *Kāśyapasaṃhitā* that a pregnant woman's actions, including her diet and social associations, can negatively affect her embryo, then it is reasonable to query the social and ethical restrictions required of women in the text. If we probe the association between the social and religious injunctions and medical data the medical compilers formulate in the work, we see that the *Kāśyapasaṃhitā*'s presentation of a creation story preceding the advent of miscarriage, which alludes to popular mythologies and mythical beings, doubtlessly carried more cultural capital than straightforward medical discourse (or chart talk). This account frames the medical definition of the issue at hand with religious rationalization that appeals to the emotions inherent to the situation as well as, if not more than, the physical hardship.

Chapter 5

The King's Disease

Like the narratives of fever and miscarriage in the previous two chapters, the ayurvedic narrative of the "king's disease" (*rājayakṣman*) that I examine in the present chapter portrays a pathology in which an ethical transgression brings about a biophysical affliction. The affliction in this case severely emaciates the body by drying up its vital fluids and attenuating its tissues. Similar to the medical story of fever, the narrative development of the king's disease begins in the divine realm after originating because of a particular deity's errant behavior and then moves to earth and the world of humanity. The change in settings redeploys the medical message of the story to relate, and in many ways conflate, the biological and socioreligious lives of human beings. Just as fever consumed the god Dakṣa because he defied his dharmic obligations as a religious sacrificer, the prototypical patient in the narrative of the king's disease, King Moon, becomes stricken with a horrible wasting disease because of his untoward actions. As we saw in the case of Dakṣa, moreover, the consequences of fever extended beyond Dakṣa's own personal well-being. In the medical narrative of Caraka's compendium, Dakṣa's improper ritual practice produced fever, and not just for himself, but for everyone in the vicinity of his ill-constructed sacrifice. Likewise, King Moon's loss of vitality from the king's disease threatens to upset the natural flow of relatedness between himself and the other celestial bodies in the night sky. This astronomic web of relatedness serves as an allegory for the complex dharmic affairs of family, society, and statecraft in classical Hinduism.

In a clearer and more direct way than the medical narratives of fever and miscarriage, the story of the king's disease evokes a sense of cosmic physiology in Āyurveda, in which ensuring long human life is contingent on the degree to which a person's well-being accords with the functioning of an ecosystem far larger than his or her own body. The main god and goddess in this story are at once divinized symbols of astral bodies of the night sky and exemplars of human behavior. The god, King Moon, goes by the following five aliases in the story: Śaśin, Candra, Soma, Aṃśumān, and Indu. The primary goddess, Rohiṇī, is a constellation (*nakṣatra*) and the daughter of the Lord of Creatures, Prajāpati.

Terminology

The term I translate as "disease" in this chapter is *yakṣma*. The Sanskrit word *yakṣman*, with a final 'n,' for many lexicographers of the nineteenth and early twentieth centuries referred to a specific sickness of the lungs. At bottom, however, both terms—*yakṣma* and *yakṣman*—mean disease or sickness, with the term *yakṣma* traditionally used as the first stem in compound lexemes, such as *yakṣmagṛhīta*, "seized with disease," and *yakṣmagrasta*, "attacked by disease." In Sanskrit literature circa the turn of the Common Era the word *yakṣma* also crops up as the second stem in two different compounds. One instance is fairly specific, *rājayakṣma*, "king's disease" or "royal disease," and the other is fairly general, *ajñātayakṣma*, "unknown disease."[1] As an independent term, the *White Yajurveda* mentions one hundred types of *yakṣma*, although, as both Jean Filliozat and Kenneth Zysk have noted in separate publications, in the pre-classical period the term *yakṣma* routinely does not signify a particular disease but is a general word for diseases that occur in both humans and cattle.[2] In his fifth century C.E. lexicographic masterwork, the *Amarakośa*, Amarasiṃha likens the term *yakṣman* to *āmaya*, *upatāpa*, *gada*, *roga*, and *vyādhi*, all of which ordinarily refer to a general state of infirmity in Āyurveda. Amarasiṃha adds that *yakṣman* usually manifests itself as emaciation (*śoṣa*) and wasting (*kṣaya*) of the body's vital fluids and tissues.[3]

Two translations of the Sanskrit compound *rāja-yakṣman* are grammatically acceptable: "king's disease" and "royal disease." Translators have often elided these renderings, however, and opted instead for descriptions that foreground the actual wasting quality of the disease mentioned by Amarasiṃha. Hence, *rājayakṣman* is called "pulmonary consumption," "phthisis," and "tuberculosis" (occasionally the adjective "royal," *rāja*, is expressed as well, resulting in "royal consumption," "royal phthisis," and so on).[4] Mario Vallauri translated *rājayakṣman* into Italian as *tisi*, which means "wasting disease."[5] Jean Filliozat related *rājayakṣman* to cachexia, which, as he put it, can refer to "an atrophy, a paralysis or even necroses . . . if it is localised in an organ."[6] A body afflicted by a consumptive disease literally wastes away, gradually losing its metabolic capacity to turn nutrients into energy. What was called consumption in the eighteenth and nineteenth centuries in North America and Europe today is generally known as tuberculosis. It is a common misnomer that consumptive disorders are strictly pulmonary, for in fact they arise in a variety of forms that may affect different areas of the body, including the lungs, spine, and brain. To translate *rājayakṣman*, at the end of the day one must work on a case-by-case basis, looking at the individual patient and symptomatology. It can, but it does not necessarily, refer to tuberculosis or consumption. For the most part, I translate *rājayakṣman* as "king's disease" in this chapter because the *rājayakṣman* narrative, which is my primary concern here, is about a certain person who gets ill, a king, as much as (if not more than) the clinical or pathological aspects of the wasting malady itself. Elsewhere in the medical literature, the wasting effects of *rājayakṣman* are discussed at length, and treatments for it are suggested. But the story of the king's disease, as we will see shortly, is first and foremost about personal cultivation and the ethical decisions individuals make in relation to others around them.

The Narrative of the King's Disease

References to and miniature versions of the narrative of the king's disease occur in the *Suśrutasaṃhitā*, *Bhelasaṃhitā*, *Aṣṭāṅgahṛdayasaṃhitā*, and *Aṣṭāṅgasaṃgrahasaṃhitā*, and there are two additional, very brief references to the narrative in the *Carakasaṃhitā*'s section on pathology (*nidānasthāna*).[7] The longest and most elaborate version of the story in the Sanskrit medical sources is in the *Carakasaṃhitā*'s section on therapeutics (*cikitsāsthāna*). In this version of the story, translated below, the story of the king's disease is presented as an oral tutorial of Ātreya Punarvasu, which he gives to his pupil Agniveśa:

> "We will now explain the treatment for the king's disease," said venerable Ātreya.
>
> The sages indeed heard the ancient story of the gods. It was about King Moon and the vice of sexual indulgence. King Moon did not take care of his body, for he was completely addicted to the constellation Rohiṇī. His semen wasted away, and his body shrunk. [Because of his dalliances with Rohiṇī] King Moon did not have sexual relations with the remaining daughters of the Lord

> of Creatures, Prajāpati. Because of this Prajāpati heaved an angry sigh, and the anger streaming from his mouth assumed a bodily form.
>
> Previously, King Moon had accepted Prajāpati's twenty-eight daughters as his wives. But he did not attend to all of them. Due to the seriousness of his disregard for his wives [other than Rohiṇī], King Moon was overcome by Prajāpati's anger, and he lost his radiance. His excess passion [for Rohiṇī] and subsequent ineffectualness [in the presence of his other wives] caused disease to settle in King Moon.
>
> With the gods and divine sages, King Moon went to Prajāpati for relief. Seeing that King Moon's intentions were good, Prajāpati was gracious. King Moon was then treated by the divine physicians, the Aśvins, and, freed from the grasp [of disease], he shone brilliantly. The Aśvins increased King Moon's vitality, and he attained pure lucidity. The words anger, disease, fever, and illness synonymously denote suffering. In earlier times, because this suffering was thought to be the king's, it was called the king's disease.
>
> The disease the Aśvins treated [in the heavens] then descended to the world of humankind. It is said that humans who catch this disease are afflicted on account of four causes: performing actions beyond one's abilities, suppression of natural urges, drying up [of the bodily fluids], and irregular diet.[8]

The fundamental premise of this narrative emerges in the third paragraph, where the history of King Moon's agreement with Prajāpati is explained. There we see that King Moon's actions clearly affect his somatic well-being, which is inextricably tied to his lunar capacities to illumine the night sky and to visit every lunar mansion on his regular orbit. His failure to uphold his conjugal commitments, therefore, disrupts his relationships with other bodies in the night sky. Moving from outer space to the ground of humankind, the narrative connects the four causes of the king's disease listed at the end of the story—performing actions beyond one's abilities, suppression of natural urges, drying up of the bodily fluids, and irregular diet—to a person's social behavior. What is more, the disorder wrought by this disease, as shown in King Moon's case, not only affects the individual actor, but it also causes collateral damage to the actor's relationships and environment. The weightiness of this lesson applies to all human beings, but especially to men. It is, moreover, a somatic lesson that applies unambiguously to the classical Indian kṣatriya king, here exemplified by King Moon, whose dharmic obligations and political power were enormous on several levels and his authority extended over many people. The king's physical well-being thus was especially important in the classical Indian world, and the classical medical sources bear this out.

Regal and Mythic History

From where does the association of royalty with a wasting disease come? What are the reasons that this medical narrative connects the king (*rāja*) to a wasting disease (*yakṣman*)? In Western cultural history, the wasting disease generally known as consumption has at times been associated with kings. Consumption had regal connotations in medieval Europe, for example, where it was commonly known as the "king's evil." Unlike the Indian context, in which kings were the prototypical patients because of their failure to attend properly to their royal duties, European monarchs were thought to possess powers capable of healing men and women who suffered from wasting diseases. The supposedly swine-borne consumptive disease, scrofula[9], for instance, was commonly perceived in medieval Europe to be a somatically manifested evil that only certain monarchs could eradicate.[10] The practice of royal healing is recorded in France as early as the fifth century C.E., performed by King Clovis, who believed (as did several of his successors) that he received from God at the time of his enthronement a bona fide power to heal the sick. In eleventh-century England, Edward the Confessor claimed a similar power for the English monarchy; even Queen Anne (reign: 1702–1714), the last of the English rulers to observe the regal curative practice, reportedly extended her healing touch to some of her scrofulous subjects. The English poet and lexicographer Samuel Johnson, at the young age of four (in 1713), was apparently among them, though reportedly he was not cured. In Hungary, King Franz Josef I's royal touch allegedly cured a sufferer of scrofula as late as 1886.[11]

In India, the story of the king's disease in ayurvedic literature—the direct opposite of the European king's evil, in that in the South Asian context the king suffers from, rather than cures, a wasting disease—likely developed out of a Ṛgvedic nuptial hymn to Soma, the Moon, and Sūryā, the daughter of the Sun. The story establishes a relationship between the Moon, the Sun and the Earth, and additionally places the Moon in the "lap" or "seat" of the constellations: "By means of Soma the Ādityas are strong; by Soma the Earth is great; thus, Soma is placed in the lap of these constellations."[12] The phrase "in the lap" refers to the Moon's heavenly orbit through the constellation-laden night sky. By the time of the *Yajurveda,* however, the Sanskrit term for "lap" (*upastha*) had come to signify human, especially female, genitalia.[13] Moreover, the constellations were regularly identified as the daughters of Prajāpati, and among them King Moon was said to be smitten most of all with Rohiṇī, Prajāpati's ninth daughter. Thus, in placing the Moon in the collective lap of the constellations, the late Vedic interpretation of the Ṛgvedic hymn came to mean that the Moon was wedded (in a connubially erotic sense) not only to the daughter of the Sun, Sūryā, but also to the daughters of Prajāpati, that is, he was also connected in a conjugal sense to the constellations of the night sky.[14]

The source from which the authors of the *Carakasaṃhitā* appear to have culled the plotline for their narrative of the king's disease is the *Taittirīyasaṃhitā,* the chief recension of the *Black Yajurveda.* In this source Prajāpati grants the hands of his thirty-three daughters in marriage to King Moon (called Soma).[15] Before long it becomes clear that Moon fancies Prajāpati's daughter Rohiṇī more than the others; this causes Rohiṇī's sisters to become upset, and they race home to their father, and beg to be released from the marriage. When Moon demands that Prajāpati send back his thirty-two other wives, Prajāpati insists that Moon promise to spend an equal amount of time with each one of his daughters. Moon agrees, and Prajāpati orders his daughters to return to Moon's abode. But Moon quickly breaks his pledge and spends all of his time with Rohiṇī. Because he breaks his vow, Moon comes down with a devastating internal disease called *yakṣma.*[16] It came to be called *rāja-yakṣma* because it afflicted the *rāja,* King Moon.

In the *Carakasaṃhitā*'s narrative, *rājayakṣman* assumes a bodily form on the winds of Prajāpati's sigh of anger. Although the authors of Caraka's compendium do not elaborate on this physical form of the disease, the description evokes the mythic origin of fever that I discussed in Chapter 3, in which fever shoots out of Rudra's third eye, destroys Dakṣa-Prajāpati's sacrifice, and heats up everyone in the area of the sacrificial grounds. Here too an affliction springs forth from the body of a god, Prajāpati, who in this sense resembles Rudra in that he manufactures the affliction. But unlike his namesake in the *Carakasaṃhitā*'s fever narrative, Dakṣa-Prajāpati, whose errant social and ritual behavior provokes Rudra's anger, which becomes fever, Prajāpati in the story of the king's disease is neither a recipient of an affliction nor the primary actor whose behavior brings an affliction into being. Instead, he breathes the king's disease into existence—"Prajāpati heaved an angry sigh, and the anger streaming from his mouth assumed a bodily form." The anthropomorphism of this disease is further developed in later Hindu mythology. The very same king's disease that Prajāpati exhales into existence in the compendium of Caraka appears and takes on a veritable life of its own in the mythology of the *Kālikā Purāṇa,* in which the ominous Rājayakṣman is married to Miss Black (Kṛṣṇā), the daughter of Death:

> Then the terrifying Yakṣman advanced from the nostrils of Dakṣa, the great-souled one, who was filled with anger. His mouth has dreadful teeth, black like charcoal. He is very tall, with very few hairs on his head. He is emaciated, with veins all over his body. After resting a while, with a stick in his hand and his face hanging down, he casts his eyes downwards, coughing, and longing for sexual pleasure with young maidens. . . .
>
> Brahmā said: "O King's Disease (Rājayakṣman)! You will dwell in the man who is always having sex with women day and night and at twilight. Into such a smarmy man, who constantly copulates with women, you should enter as catarrh, asthma, and cough. Miss Black, daughter of Death, whose qualities are suitable to you, is your wife and constant companion."[17]

The somatic lesson that excessive sexual activity with multiple partners leads to physiologic dysfunction and potential erasure of a man's virility is unmistakable, not to mention more attention grabbing, in the *Kālikā Purāṇa*'s anthropomorphized illustration of the king's disease as Rājayakṣman. Sexually predacious men, the *Kālikā Purāṇa* seems to suggest, do not just contract the king's disease, they actually transform into the disease, literally becoming the myth's ill-omened figure, Rājayakṣman. Wreaking bodily havoc from the inside out, the disease starts as a cough, asthma, or catarrh and ends with the ultimate death knell: the *rājayakṣman*-ed man's marriage to death's daughter, Miss Black (Kṛṣṇā).

Astral and Terrestrial Observations

The wasting away of King Moon, that is, his experience of the king's disease, is initially set in the context of the lunar orbit, and it is specifically linked to Moon's neglect of the various constellations to which he is married. Drawing out the astrological and marital homologies, the constellation-wives represent the lunar mansions in which King Moon is supposed to tarry throughout his monthly orbit. Each night, Moon enters (has sex with) a different lunar mansion (wife), thus completing his calendrical (nuptial) obligations. Where variations of this story occur in Sanskrit literature, the sources differ on how many of Prajāpati's daughters King Moon actually married (which is also to say that the sources disagree on the number of constellations situated along the lunar orbit). Usually the number is either twenty-seven or twenty-eight, the latter of which we find in the *Carakasaṃhitā*; in the *Taittirīyasaṃhitā*, as we saw above, there were thirty-three.

Irrespective of the number of wives King Moon had, in every variation of the story he becomes especially obsessed with Rohiṇī. He ultimately spends most of his time with her on his orbital gambol, and for this reason he neglects his other wives. David White has discussed the important astrophysical activities implied by the *Taittirīyasaṃhitā*'s depiction of King Moon's tryst with Rohiṇī, his subsequent affliction with the king's disease, and the eventual treatment of his disease. The same cosmic implications to which White draws our attention, I suggest, are present in the *Carakasaṃhitā*'s variant of the older *Taittirīyasaṃhitā* narrative. White explains:

> It is here that Candra [the Moon], at that point at which he is "closest to the sun," spends himself completely in the clutches of his starry wife [Rohiṇī], and the moon disappears. His *rasa*, his vigor, his semen completely dried up, the moon must perform a *soma* (which is both a name for and the stuff of the moon, the *rasa* par excellence) sacrifice in order to recover his lost *rasa*, and so the cycle begins anew.[18]

The point in which the Moon is "closest to the sun" is the twenty-ninth day of the monthly lunar cycle. On this day, the moon is directly between the sun and the earth. The side of the moon facing the sun is lighted by the sun's light, while the side facing the earth is completely dark so that the moon is invisible to the earth at this juncture (with the rare exception, of course, of a solar eclipse whereby the disc of the moon moves entirely in front of the sun so that all light from the sun going to earth is temporarily blocked). This is called a New Moon. The sacrifice White refers to is the offering prescribed in the *Taittirīyasaṃhitā* to treat a person "seized by an evil disease" (*pāpayakṣmagṛhīta*). It consists of an offering to the Ādityas, and it should be offered at the time of the New Moon.[19] Additionally,

White has shown that the story of Moon's orbit forms a connection between the height of the Indian hot season and the king's disease. The connection lies, he argues, in the desiccative effects of the sun and its fire and the moon and its fluid, the most important fluid of which is the moon's *rasa*, the mythological homologue of which is King Moon's semen:

> Here the parallel, between the fiery (*āgneya*) and the lunar (*saumya*) semesters of the year on the one hand, and the waning and the waxing fortnights of the lunar month on the other, is transparently evident. In both cases, that half of a temporal cycle characterized by desiccation (of the ecosystem, of the moon's *rasa*) is associated with the heat of the sun and death. Royal consumption is most likely to occur at the end of the solar semester, just as the disappearance of King Moon occurs at the end of the dark fortnight during which he has dissipated himself by exposing himself to the draining heat of the sexual embrace of the starry woman Rohiṇī. King Moon's loss of *rasa* is manifested in the latter half of his monthly cycle, by the waning of the moon, by its diminution, by one digit (*kalā*) on each succeeding night. And, at the end of its dark fortnight, the moon, completely dissipated, disappears.[20]

King Moon's vital fluids severely dissipate in the waning half of his orbital rounds, when he visits his favorite wife, Rohiṇī, and uses up his semen completely. But he recovers during the waxing half of every month. White's analysis of the story of the king's disease, although immensely helpful for its literary and historical insight, is only partially useful to the present study. At the end of the day, his analysis primarily concerns the later half of King Moon's orbit, his rejuvenation (*rasāyana*) following his emaciation, not the pathology (*nidāna*) of the illness and the collateral repercussions that could ensue if King Moon is not rejuvenated, which are my main interests here.

The moon regenerates each month, and its rasa returns with the monthly *soma* sacrifice with the monthly *soma* sacrifice. The moon's monthly wax and wane is a constant occurrence in the night sky, provided that humans perform the *soma* sacrifice during the moon's waning phase. There is a clear homological relationship established here between lunar activity and human sacrificial activity, between the astral and terrestrial orders of the cosmos. The macrocosmic waxings and wanings of the moon are mirrored and motivated by the microcosmic sacrifice. When properly aligned, they jointly maintain the overarching, universal order or truth, known from the Vedic period onward by the principle of *ṛta*. But what does this cosmological reading mean for the narrative of the king's disease in the compendium of Caraka, which is, after all, about the manifestation of this wasting disease among humanity? The lunation cycle is quite regular, going from new moon to full moon and back to new moon again every month. Over the past half decade or so, it has been fashionable in popular culture and new age circles to hear claims that this cycle illustrates the monthly menses of premenopausal women, the phases of the moon paralleling the buildup, shedding, and re-buildup of a woman's menstrual fluids. The idea that women can align their menstruation cycles according to the phases of the moon and thereby manage their reproduction according to the lunar schedule is a technique Louise Lacey famously called "lunaception" in 1975, and it has been popular in North America ever since.[21] This notion has of course been around a lot longer than Lacey's observations, and it has existed in many societies other than the United States. But have men ever been thought to have a similar, lunar-based physiologic cycle associated with their reproductive fluids? The *Carakasaṃhitā*'s narrative could be read to suggest that in fact they do have a parallel to the female menstrual cycle. Casual observation, however, would suggest that no, they do not. After ejaculation, men recover their semen very quickly in comparison to the length of the lunar cycle. Also, unlike the menstrual cycles of women, which last roughly a month, men may go for long periods of time, far longer than a calendar month in some cases, without shedding their seed. To be sure, in numerous Sanskrit works, from the Upaniṣads through the Purāṇas, the retention of semen over spans of time far beyond one month is thought to bring about enormous mental clarity and preternatural powers. On account of this conception, we find in Sanskrit literature the image of the "pregnant yogi" who has stockpiled great powers within himself by retaining his semen.[22]

The *Suśrutasaṃhitā* contains a passage on the growth and regeneration of semen in the male body that is useful to the present discussion of male potency. The original source of a man's semen, the text states, is rasa. Rasa is also the source of menstrual fluid in women.[23] In Āyurveda, rasa is a fiery "nourishing juice" that is metabolized from food and circulates throughout the body after digestion. Out of rasa, the six other bodily substances (*dhātus*) are formed and sustained, developing in the following order according to the compendium of Suśruta: "From the nourishing juice comes blood, and from that comes flesh. From flesh comes fat. From fat comes bone, and from that comes marrow. From marrow comes semen."[24] Further along in Suśruta's compendium it is said that rasa spends 3,015 *kalās* (at about 2.35 minutes per *kalā*) in each bodily tissue. In the *Ṛgveda*, where we find the earliest attestations of *kalā*, the term signified a sixteenth portion of any whole unit. Slightly later, a lunar association is applied to *kalā* as a unit of time measurement aligned with the sixteen digits of the moon.[25] The total amount of time it takes for a body's rasa to produce semen in men and menstrual fluid in women is one lunar month, or approximately 18,090 *kalās* (roughly 29.5 days or 6 bodily tissues at 3,015 *kalās* per tissue).[26] Not unlike the menstrual cycle of women, then, save the regular pouring out of fluids, in the estimation of the compilers of the *Suśrutasaṃhitā*, a man has a monthly seminal cycle. The basic physiologic problem of the king's disease, the commentator Cakrapāṇidatta calculated, is that it causes an obstruction of rasa, thus depriving the body's tissues of their "nourishing juice" and retarding or occluding the production of semen in men and menstrual fluids in women.[27] At a cosmic level, just as the performance of the *soma* sacrifice ensures that the moon recovers the cool unctuosity (its *soma*) lost during its waning phases, likewise ayurvedic medicine (including diet and potency medicines, which fall under the ayurvedic branch of *vājīkaraṇa*), can facilitate the metabolic flow of the highly nutritive rasa to ensure the production of semen according to a regular monthly schedule.[28]

Piggybacking on the physiologic lesson, the medical narrative of the king's disease provides another somatic lesson, but of a decidedly ethical nature, which is designed to curb the man-about-town's overindulgence in sexual activity. Licentious men can and do act like King Moon acts in the story, dispensing their seed in one fell swoop, and often when and where they should not dispense it. The ethical lesson, just as in the previous two chapters, is about personal cultivation and behaviors that people—in this case men—choose to perform despite clear knowledge of religious responsibility and social expectations that ought to lead them to act otherwise. The story of the king's disease is about the dharma of men and husbands in relation to the people they regularly relate to on a physical level, specifically women and wives. What is more, by positing King Moon as the prototypical patient of the king's disease, the narrative's authors also focus on the dharma of the kṣatriya king, who throughout Indian history typically had several wives at one time and whose socioethical commitments to other people—his subjects, court advisors, allies, tutelary deities, and so forth—were many and significant. The lesson here is that for men in general and especially kings, a healthy male body can quickly become the site of affliction if a man's behavior aligns with the medical tradition's classification of reprehensibility. Moreover, a man's afflicted body will inexorably disrupt not only his own life and medical well-being but also the flow of relatedness between himself and the bodies of others around him.

The excessive sexual appetite of King Moon in the *Carakasaṃhitā*'s medical narrative belongs to a fairly long-established association in India between a man's loss of vitality and the drying up of his most vital fluid, semen. The compendium of Caraka itself says that the wasting disease of *rājayakṣman* arose because King Moon lost his semen. I have translated the word "semen" from the Sanskrit word *sneha*, following Cakrapāṇidatta's gloss: "[B]y the word *sneha* the essential elements semen (*śukra*) and vitality (*ojas*) are meant."[29] What exactly is "vitality," *ojas*? G. Jan Meulenbeld has traced the lexical changes in the meaning of the Sanskrit word *ojas* from its Vedic meaning of a "force" inherent to the gods to its physiologic meaning of a "fluid substance, a constituent of all human beings, both male and female."[30] Meticulously tracing the textual occurrences of *ojas* in Sanskrit medical and non-medical literatures, he has shown the high degree of variability and divergent use of the concept in ayurvedic history. The term, moreover, has several meanings in contemporary Āyurveda that it did not have in the classical or medieval periods. In the end, Meulenbeld asks whether the term *ojas*, because it has been so radically divorced from its apparent original usages, should be dropped altogether as un-ayurvedic rather than continue to serve the needs of the day.[31] Notwithstanding Meulenbeld's useful query about the contemporary use of classical medical terminology, if we stick to the classical sources and their commentators, we can arrive at a fairly specific understanding of what Cakrapāṇidatta had in mind when he was reading the *Carakasaṃhitā* in the eleventh century. Citing the *Suśrutasaṃhitā*, Cakrapāṇidatta states that *ojas* is not a thing. It is the quintessence of the seven bodily tissues and the vital "force that supports life."[32] Semen is the substantive means, the veritable vehicle for King Moon's vitality (*ojas*). After completely expelling his semen during his stopover in Rohiṇī's lunar mansion, King Moon did not have enough punch to light up the night sky, an inability, it seems, that prevented him from finishing his orbital rounds with his other wives.

The term Cakrapāṇidatta takes as semen, *sneha*, generally means "oiliness" or "viscidity." He noted only the medical application of the term, however. In Sanskrit dramatic and poetic texts, *sneha* also frequently means "affection" and "love." The double meaning is highly relevant here in the dramatization of a medical issue. It is clear in the story that King Moon's dalliances with Rohiṇī entail sexual activity. For it is during his time with Rohiṇī that he uses up his semen, and for that he loses his vitality. His involvement with Rohiṇī effectively renders him incapable of having sexual relations with his other twenty-six wives (or twenty-seven or thirty-two, depending on the source), and consequently he shows them no love or affection. By overindulging with Rohiṇī only, King Moon used up all of his *sneha*. Sans *sneha*, King Moon could mete out neither the sexual fluid nor his love and affection, which a husband is obliged to impart to his wives (or, at least in this story, he cannot deliver the physical and emotional *sneha* that his wives would like him to deliver). In Hindu mythology, the moon is often associated with dharma, particularly, as Jan Gonda observed, as a "witness who sees whether men observe the rules of dharma."[33] In Chapter 3, I explained how the *Carakasaṃhitā* drew connections between physical and moral decline in the narrative of fever. In the narrative of the king's disease we find a similar framework. The first person attacked by the desiccative disease *rājayakṣman* is King Moon. What is the reason his body wastes away? He is portrayed as blameworthy for a moral transgression. Yet unlike his historically characteristic role of witnessing the auspicious and inauspicious dharmic activity of humankind, here Moon is not a moral authority but an anti-model. He presents a somatic lesson to be learned via negativa, in that he is the exemplar from whom human men and kings learn how not to act in the world.

Before I turn to the paradigmatic patient in this medical narrative, the king, a word about method may be useful here. The type of medical hermeneutics that I am elaborating in this book recognizes portions of the literature—an ayurvedic narrative tradition, or tradition of medical storytelling in Āyurveda—that has until now gone unstudied in the history of Indian medicine. Methodologically, I am also presenting a somewhat novel way to read the Sanskrit medical classics, which suggests the compilers of classical Āyurveda had an expansive awareness of Indian textual corpora and knowledge systems outside of what is traditionally classified as medicine. The authors of classical Āyurveda were highly skilled vaidyas and educators, of course, whose chart talk stands as the prototypical literary expression of the tradition. Yet the intertextual complexity of the medical narratives in the Sanskrit sources also demonstrates that diverse avenues of literary expression were utilized and that the ideology of Āyurveda was seen to extend into numerous cultural domains, such as religion and social construction, where, crucially, the medical authors underscored the fundamental importance of somatic health to the success of religious practice and social welfare. A thorough documentation of this multilayered "medical" knowledge is enormously useful to understand the cultural location of Āyurveda in Indian history, and it adds to our understanding of the interaction and transmission of Sanskrit scientific knowledge systems in general. Recognizing, for example, that a Vedic concept like macrocosmic-microcosmic accord (*ṛta*) perdures in the sources of Āyurveda, and explaining how the ayurvedic authors made use of the concept, we can begin to appreciate the demonstrably active role that Āyurveda played in the preservation, reworking, and transmission of Indian cultural knowledge.

The Royal Patient

The *Carakasaṃhitā* asserts that the king's disease arises in humans because of one of four causes: overexertion, suppression of natural urges, drying up of the body's vital fluids, and poor diet. King Moon's health changes from fine to awful in the *rājayakṣman* narrative because of the third cause. He was sapped of his vital fluids, especially his semen (*śukra*). In this sense, the king's disease is indeed a consumptive disease, although not necessarily tuberculosis, phthisis, or consumption. It is simply, as Mario Vallauri had it, a wasting disease.

The pathology of the king's disease in this medical narrative is primarily about the essence or the nature of being human. The narrative's central somatic lesson pertains less to abnormal anatomic or physiologic conditions that promote somatic wasting and more to modal states and patterns of relationships in the specific people the disease targets, namely, men in general and kings in particular. Francis Zimmermann has argued that the mythological literature associated with the king's disease teaches us that when people abandon their dharma and fall into self-destructive behavior, they often are susceptible to a great deal more than just biological illness. A person can slip, Zimmermann writes, into "a consumption or dessication [sic] of his existence, a sort of ontological disease, one which we would be mistaken to reduce flatly to phthisis."[34] As an ontological disease, *rājayakṣman* is therefore not merely the king's disease; it is the king disease or the king of diseases, in that, as the *Carakasaṃhitā* reports, *rājayakṣman* is the "most pernicious of all diseases."[35] It depletes the body's fluids and wastes away the body's tissues, slowly and painfully erasing altogether a person's entire existence.

In the narrative in Caraka's compendium, King Moon is a metaphor, primarily for the human male but also for the kṣatriya, or warrior-king. The ontological pathology of the king's disease translates from one realm—the heavens and King Moon's interstellar love affairs—to another—the earth and the responsibilities of the male protector, the warrior-king. Just as King Moon lost his physical vitality after a chain of morally questionable deeds (and non-deeds), the king who neglects his dharmic duties to serve and protect his subjects and his land by following a base urge like lust will be saddled with the king's disease. This is no small issue in the ancient Indian context. The kṣatriya king in Indian history was thought to be semi-divine. He was, as Sheldon Pollock put it, "no simple god or man but an intermediate, combinatory being that draws from and transcends the powers of both realms."[36] Depictions of the king as a god on earth can be found in numerous genres and throughout various periods of Sanskrit literature. But this twofold description is perhaps nowhere clearer than in the two Indian epics, the *Rāmāyaṇa* and the *Mahābhārata*. The *Rāmāyaṇa* states in no uncertain terms: "It is kings—make no mistake about it—who confer righteous merit, something so hard to acquire, and precious life itself. One must never harm them, never criticize, insult, or oppose them. Kings are gods who walk the earth in the form of men."[37] In the *Mahābhārata*, men of the Kaurava and Pāṇḍava families are frequently called *narendra*, "Indra of Men" (Indra being *devendra*, "King of Gods").[38] Because the divine and human worlds were thought to be ruled according to the same cosmic laws, in the *Mahābhārata* the kṣatriya king is looked to as the basis and guardian of order on earth to the same degree that Indra is looked to as the basis and guardian of order in the heavens.[39] But the medical literature is quick to remind us that the divine nature of earthly kings is neither eternal nor complete. Authority varies as a king's human qualities change over time. Like all human beings, human kings too are subject to disease and death.

The correlation between the cosmic and the terrestrial monarchs established by the medical narrative of the king's disease is appropriately grand. In addition to his divine status on earth, from very early on in Indian history the king is depicted as the nucleus of human society, largely because of his vital role as sacrificer-in-chief. Through his role as the promoter and funder of the sacrifice, the king embodies the annual recreation of the universe and recalibration of the earth and its peoples with the heavens and the gods.[40] Much of the classical ayurvedic literature integrated the customary Indian view of the king as the Mount Meru of human society, upon whom the health of every human body depends.[41] The somatic well-being of the king, therefore, was paramount to the compilers of the Sanskrit medical classics, in which, following Zimmermann's observations, the king is "the most important of all patients, *the king is the patient par excellence*, because his state of health expresses the *artha* (well-being) of all his subjects."[42] Biophysical misfortune for the king essentially augurs misfortune for every person who counts on him for protection and sustenance. The *Suśrutasaṃhitā* even devotes an entire chapter to the health of the king.[43]

A king's primary dharmic duties in the Dharmaśāstra literature are, in sum, to govern without tyrannizing, to battle bravely and honorably, and eventually to die a heroic death.[44] Albeit just the basics of the duties of the ancient Indian regent, this three-part summary nicely spells out the king's central role as supreme sacrificer, not simply as the religious sacrificer (*yajamāna*) but as the person in society who must constantly give of himself for everyone who lives in his kingdom.[45] Again, the *Mahābhārata* is an excellent source on this subject. There we learn on numerous occasions that members of the kṣatriya class, the warrior-kings, routinely pride themselves on their propensity to give rather than receive.[46] Such boasting stems from a desire not to appear needful or in any way without resources, like a beggar whose sustenance comes not from his or her own life and potency but rather depends on the charity of others. The classical medical tradition describes this power dichotomy—to beg or to give—in physiologic terms. A healthy person has the ability to give him- or herself fully to his or her dharma, whereas a sick person is hindered in this endeavor. The foremost determinants of physiologic health, according to the classical Sanskrit sources, are the body's vital fluids. When the fluids dry up, the body languishes and becomes ineffectual as an instrument to accomplish the duties, or dharmas, entailed by a person's life station in society. A king without semen—the human homologue of the lunar *soma* and the embodiment of a man's vitality (*ojas*)—is a king without his crown, so to speak, and in this way he is no different from any other male commoner. His kingdom is moribund because he is effectively impotent as a ruler and warrior.

To reestablish King Moon's emaciated and wasted body, the *Carakasaṃhitā*'s narrative explains that the Aśvins restored his vitality, which in turn brought about "pure lucidity" (*śuddhaṃ sattvam*). In his commentary on this phrase, Cakrapāṇidatta equates "lucidity" (*sattva*) with "mind" (*manas*).[47] His reading is instructive. The replenishment of King Moon's vitality boosts his intellectual capacity, rendering him mentally able to realize his dharma as the earth's moon. He quickly knows he must stop spending so much time with the constellation Rohiṇī, resume his orbital journey, and, in so doing, cool off the earth following the solar dehydration of the hot season. For the human king, the replenishment of his vitality gives him purity of mind to resume his dharmic obligation to look after the welfare of his subjects, kingdom, and family.

Sex is not the only reason the *Carakasaṃhitā* states a man's semen, and thus his vitality, may run out, however. It is one cause of the body's wasting, but not the only cause. Some of the most severe cases of *rājayakṣman* arise because of psychological stress, as Caraka's compendium explains in a passage shortly after the narrative of the king's disease: "[S]emen and vitality decrease because of envy, yearning, fear, anxiety, anger, grief, overexertion, excessive sexual intercourse, and fasting."[48] On this view, the connection between purity of mind and possession of vitality is patently clear. What is good for oneself is self-knowledge. Who am I? What are my abilities? Where do I stand, and what are my responsibilities in relation to those around me and to my environment?[49] To answer these questions, one needs mental clarity. To think clearly, one needs energy. It might come as a surprise that the *Carakasaṃhitā* recommends inward-focused action (*nivṛtti*) as a chief means for "causing a well-nourished condition" (*puṣṭikarāṇa*), the very antithesis of the emaciation wrought on a body by the king's disease.[50] It is surprising because the discussion is about kings, and activity focused inwardly, *nivṛtti*, would seem to be a recipe for a regent's ruin at the hands of either his own people or external invaders. That said, the term *puṣṭikarāṇa*, "causing a well-nourished condition," may also mean simply "causing plumpness," in which case the absence of activity sometimes associated with the concept *nivṛtti* could produce the opposite condition of emaciation, that is, the fleshy rotundity that comes from the abandonment of outward-focused activity (*pravṛtti*).

In Āyurveda, the concept of inward-focused action—*nivṛtti*—stands in opposition to outward-focused action—*pravṛtti*. Addressing this opposition, the *Carakasaṃhitā*'s message is demonstrative: "The root of this [world] and of all afflictions is *pravṛtti*; *nivṛtti* is the cessation [of them]. It is said that *pravṛtti* is suffering and *nivṛtti* is happiness. That truth begets knowledge."[51] The term *pravṛtti* literally means turning outward and moving forth. It is a principle used to describe a person's worldly and socially engaged endeavors, and it relates to things such as social relationships and religious enterprises. It is the natural condition of sentient creatures. Yet *pravṛtti* is also the source of every misery. The outward-focused action inherent to human nature drives the karmic process of cause and effect that ensures the ongoing cycle (*saṃsāra*) of rebirth and redeath. Conversely, *nivṛtti* literally means turning inward, and returning. It is a principle that often entails asceticism, celibacy, and withdrawal from the world of social and economic relationships. *Nivṛtti* is a source of happiness, for a disciplined, contemplative life involving ascetic withdrawal has since the time of the early Upaniṣads been thought to minimize the effects of one's karmic debt; this in turn may have the effect of, in the long run, permanently releasing one from saṃsāra or, at the very least, ensuring an enjoyable present lifetime.[52]

The discussion of the principles of *pravṛtti* and *nivṛtti*, especially concerning when, and to what degree, the kṣatriya king in Indian society should turn his attention outward and/or inward, continues in the next chapter on the allegory *The Joy of Life* (*Jīvānandanam*). This text stands as the acme of narrative medical discourse in Sanskrit literature, and in many ways it marks the height of narrativizing the body and the medical patient in the history of Indian medicine.

Chapter 6

The Joy of Life of Ānandarāyamakhin

Medical narratives in Indian medical literature both reflect and direct social perceptions of disease. This is perhaps nowhere more evident than in Ānandarāyamakhin's (hereafter Ānandarāya) seven-act allegory, *The Joy of Life* (*Jīvānandanam*). As in Chapter 5, in this chapter the king's disease is central to the discussion, for the personification of *rājayakṣman*, King Disease, along with his afflictive martial cohort threatens to destroy the hero of Ānandarāya's play, King Life. But unlike Chapter 5, *The Joy of Life* is an allegory, and its account of the assault of King Disease on the body of King Life unfolds simultaneously on two parallel levels, a somatic level and a social level. Each character in the play at once represents a part of the human body and an actor in an imperial Indian society. The play conveys the basic but perspicacious vision that the physiology of an individual body affects, communicates with, and is under the influence of the larger social physiology of its surroundings. The result is a collision of physiologies, so to speak, and in the play King Life must learn to manage the welfare of his body and royal court amid the often-deleterious world around him. Endemic to the human condition, in other words, there is an ongoing series of collisions between an individual and society. How people act in the world and negotiate these confrontations affects their physical well-being. This is precisely the lesson King Life learns in the play, for the well-being of his body and royal court is contingent on the ways in which he engages with and/or disengages from the affairs around him.

The Joy of Life in Context

Around the turn of the seventeenth and eighteenth centuries in Thanjavur, south India (Tamil Nadu), Ānandarāya composed *The Joy of*

Life as a stage-piece. It débuted during the reign of the Maratha king Śāhajī (Śhahujī in Marathi), who either ascended to the Thanjavur throne in 1683 following the death of his father, Venkojī, the first Maratha ruler of Thanjavur (and younger half-brother of the famous Maratha ruler, Śivajī) or, following the *Dharmakuṭa* (a commentary on the *Rāmāyaṇa*), he took the throne after Venkojī abdicated the Thanjavur regency in 1684. Śāhajī ruled Thanjavur until his death on 28 September 1711.[1]

There has been some disagreement about the authorship of *The Joy of Life*.[2] A handful of scholars have recognized someone named Vedakavi as the author of the work.The proponents of this argument, however, have not sufficiently explained why the text should be ascribed to Vedakavi rather than Ānandarāya. Apparently following the lead of Kuppuswami Sastri, who made the assertion of Vedakavi's authorship first, the argument is that Ānandarāya was Vedakavi's patron.[3] The Sanskrit text itself does not support this assertion, however. Indeed, the name Vedakavi is not mentioned in the work. Rather, the text clearly states that the play (*nāṭaka*) was written or created (*praṇīta*) by Ānandarāya.[4] What is more, as I show below, in the play's introduction the stage manager (*sūtradhāra*) declares to his assistant that the poet (*kavi*) of *The Joy of Life* is Ānandarāyamakhin. Although future text-historical research on *The Joy of Life* may reveal an association between Ānandarāya and someone named Vedakavi in Maratha-era Thanjavur, it is beyond the scope of the present treatment of narrative medicine to take up the debate concerning Ānandarāya's authorship here.[5] Using Duraiswami Aiyangar's English introduction and Sanskrit *bhūmikā* to the 1947 Adyar Library edition of the text, we also glean some information about Ānandarāya's life. For example, we learn that he came from a family of gifted scholars, playwrights, artists, and court officials. In his own right, Ānandarāya was a veritable factotum in the Thanjavur court of Śāhajī, serving at once as a "chancellor, house-priest, spiritual advisor and court poet."[6]

It appears that Ānandarāya composed *The Joy of Life* as both an entertainment and pedagogical piece for the Bṛhadīśvara Temple festival in Thanjavur, with the general intention of conveying knowledge about medicine (Āyurveda), dharma, and devotional Hinduism (bhakti). Each of these themes is expressed and explained in the play through direct quotations and paraphrases of important Sanskrit works, such as the *Arthaśāstra*, *Bhagavadgītā*, *Rāmāyaṇa*, poetic and purāṇic works, and the big and little trios of Āyurveda. Working in 1937, the translator of *The Joy of Life* into German, Adolf Weckerling, argued that the basic ideology of the play is religion, particularly Śaiva devotionalism. More recently, Maria Schetelich has suggested that Ānandarāya's play is primarily a meditation on royal authority and leadership.[7] Mario Vallauri, who translated *The Joy of Life* into Italian in 1929, offered the best assessment of the play's thematic coverage, noting that instead of privileging one area over another, it appears that Ānandarāya was interested in demonstrating the complementarity of traditional Indian knowledge concerning medical theories about somatic care, religious practice, and civic responsibility in the everyday lives of citizens living in Thanjavur and the Maratha kingdom.[8] I agree with Vallauri, and would suggest that Ānandarāya's play offers many literary innovations that are reflective and very much a part of the wave of intense Sanskrit productivity in the two centuries before British colonialism on the Indian subcontinent (ca. 1550–1750), when Indian thinkers reformulated scientific genres and developed cross-disciplinary scholarly writing.[9] Remarkably, to date *The Joy of Life* has received very little attention from historians of Indian medicine and scholars of Sanskrit literature from the early-modern period in Indian history. Ānandarāya's play is a very rich interdisciplinary piece, as well as a valuable contribution to the history of Sanskrit allegorical writing, from this important and vibrant literary era.

I also would like to suggest that Vallauri's evenhanded analysis of *The Joy of Life* runs the risk of missing the emphasis on medicine in Ānandarāya's work, which always lies beneath the allusions and direct references to the cultural categories of religion and politics in the text. In particular, in this play Ānandarāya makes the critical observation that in order to be a successful ruler, a productive citizen, and a religious votary a person needs first to attend to the well-being of his or her body. The themes of politics and religion are indeed present in the play; in many ways they are presented not as distinct cultural categories but instead as intertwined ideologies that direct people's personal decisions and social activities. The themes of religious devotion and practice, however, support rather than determine the play's fundamental messages, which are first and foremost somatic lessons of a medical order. The themes of statecraft and politics represent the duty (or dharma) of the play's hero, King Life, to which he must attend, but it is a secondary obligation to be pursued after he cares for his body, the cultivation of which is his primary duty—which is, in other words, King Life's body dharma.

The fact that roughly a millennium and a half separates the composition of *The Joy of Life* and the classical Sanskrit sources that I have treated in the previous chapters of this book warrants a few remarks before I proceed. There are three primary reasons for including Ānandarāya's text in the present study. First, *The Joy of Life* was composed for live performance at the Bṛhadīśvara (Śiva) Temple festival. It is the only existing piece of Sanskrit medical literature that was clearly intended for mass consumption, apparently to educate and entertain the public on matters of health and illness through drama. The medical narratives of classical Āyurveda, too, appear to have been meant for public audiences, but they do not plainly state why or how they were actually used. That Ānandarāya intended the play to be a performance piece, and that the content of the play has unambiguous medical import, suggest that the practice of narrativizing the body for medical purposes was known in Indian history. From this, we may posit that the narratives in the classical works, too, could have been designed for medical instruction. This relatively late medical text, in other words, offers us significant data to make sense of the function of medical narratives and storytelling in the classical Sanskrit medical treatises. Second, the antihero of the play, King Disease (Rājayakṣman), is a personification of the illness discussed in Chapter 5. Ānandarāya's character represents a unique stage in the imagination and narrativization of the disease in Indian medicine. A dramatic rendering of Rājayakṣman and other characters in *The Joy of Life* shows that some of the big themes of classical medical knowledge—illness (*yakṣman, roga*), life (*āyus*), health (*svāsthya, ārogya*), the body (*śarīra*), ātman—were not limited to the medical field but, historically, received attention across various Indian knowledge systems. Third, this play is a useful stepping-stone to move from the classical and medieval to modern Sanskrit-based medical traditions in India. Ānandarāya's dramatization of premodern ayurvedic literature underscores the importance of situating medicine in relation to diverse institutions and knowledge systems of Indian society. His play constructs Āyurveda as a proper foundation of culture, moreover, and helps to make sense of the many ways in which socioreligious thought informs conceptions of illness and treatments of the body in the teaching and practice of contemporary Sanskrit-based medicine in India and throughout South Asia.

Ānandarāya worked in a literary medium, allegory, that had a well-established history prior to *The Joy of Life*. But the formal academic study, or literary criticism, of allegory in Sanskrit literature, compared to metaphor (*rūpaka*) for example, is a relatively recent pursuit. It will be useful here, therefore, to consider briefly the literary genealogy to which *The Joy of Life* belongs. The English term allegory comes from the Greek *allēgoria*, which literally means veiled or figurative langauge and often refers to an extended use of metaphor. As a literary genre, allegory consists of outwardly pointing to a target, known as the primary level of signification, while simultaneously communicating a secondary order of signification. Traditional Sanskrit poetics recognizes these two levels of meaning with the terms *abhidhā* for primary meaning and *lakṣaṇa* or *guṇavāda* for secondary or metaphorical meaning. Proponents of *dhvani*-theory ("suggestion") posited yet a third level, distinct from the secondary level, called "implication" (*vyañjanā*), which they regarded as emblematic of poetic language use. This is all to say, in very short order, that the study of language ornamentation (*alaṃkāra*), or Sanskrit rhetoric, is a major, long-established, and nuanced area of scholarship on the Indian subcontinent. Yet, allegory as it is treated in the West, in which two complete stories exist simultaneously as parallel narrative trajectories, appears to be a much more modern object of scrutiny in Sanskrit poetics. For example, in a 1962 Ph.D. dissertation submitted to Agra University, Saroja Agravāla fashioned the Hindi phrases *rūpak nāṭak*, "metaphorical drama," and *rūpak pātr*, "metaphorical character" (derived from the Sanskrit phrases *rūpakanāṭaka* and *rūpakapātra*), to describe the genre and dramatis personæ in Kṛṣṇamiśra's eleventh-century allegorical work, the *Prabodhacandrodaya*.[10] More recently, Matthew Kapstein has suggested the Sanskrit neologism *pratīkanāṭaka*, "symbolic drama," has been used to categorize Vedāntadeśika's fourteenth-century allegorical opus, the *Saṃkalpasūryodaya*.[11] Although the *Prabodhacandrodaya* is the earliest known sustained allegorical drama in Sanskrit, Kṛṣṇamiśra was not the first writer of Sanskrit to use allegorical techniques.

Allegorization occurs in Sanskrit literature from very early on. The *Śvetāśvatara Upaniṣad* (4.6–7) and the *Muṇḍaka Upaniṣad* (3.1), for example, allegorize the story of the two birds in Book 1 of the *Ṛgveda* (1.164.20) to represent the opposing notions of materiality and spirit (or *prakṛti* and *puruṣa*). In his *Kuvalayānandakārikā*, Appaya Dīkṣita called this type of one-for-one equation *samāsokti*, "abbreviated speech," to denote the literary act of describing something present (the birds) while conveying a message about an abstraction or something not present (*prakṛti* and *puruṣa*).[12] This "trope of abbreviation," *samāsokti*, involves the implicit characterization of something to be signified while explicitly describing only the literal source. It is a brief or isolated tactic in Sanskrit poetics, however, not a structural feature with which to describe an entire narrative.[13] Around the first to second centuries C.E., we find allegorization in the fragments of Aśvaghoṣa's *Buddhacarita* with the three characters, Fame (Kīrti), Firmness (Dhṛti), and Wisdom (Buddhi). In the ninth century C.E., Jayanta Bhaṭṭa (author of the *Nyāyamañjari*) wrote a highly didactic and philosophical play with plenty of allegorical ornamentation, the *Āgamaḍambara*. After Kṛṣṇamiśra's *Prabodhacandrodaya*, other Sanskrit allegories appeared, such as Yaśapāla's *Mohaparājaya*, Karṇapūra's *Caitanyacandrodaya*, and two works attributed to Ānandarāya, the *Jīvānandanam* (*The Joy of Life*) and the *Vidyāpariṇayam* (*The Nuptials of Knowledge*).

Why opt for allegory to convey complex interrelationships between cultural domains like religion, politics, and medicine and, as I discuss later in this chapter, a fundamental ontological dichotomy like *pravṛtti-nivṛtti*? Allegory, after all, is a somewhat inelegant literary medium. Matthew Kapstein recently argued that allegory "suffers from the constraint of its major premise, for it must tell a story that is in fact a second story, a double task restricting the author's free creation and often lending to allegorical works a rigid, contrived quality."[14] Although it is true that handicaps are inherent to the genre, and contrivances do abound in Ānandarāya's work, where Kapstein sees a restriction of creativity in allegory I see in *The Joy of Life* the labor of a dramatist who succeeds to a remarkable degree both to entertain and elucidate abstract scholastic subjects. In the required multitasking of the genre, Ānandarāya thrives and tells not just a second story, but actually three stories—a medical story, a political story, and a religious story. He undergirds them all with the ingenious observation that the felly holding together the polythetic spokes of the human cultural wheel is a course of action—*vṛtti*—that every person forges in the world. Indeed, Ānandarāya appears to be freer creatively in this text, in which he interweaves lessons from Āyurveda, Nītiśāstra, and bhakti literature, than in his other allegory, *The Nuptials of Knowledge* (*Vidyāpariṇayam*), in which he is clearly constrained by the tradition of the nondualist philosophy of Advaita Vedānta.[15]

The Narrative Trajectory of *The Joy of Life*

Among the many members of King Life's royal retinue, the principal actors are Life's wife, Queen Reason (Buddhi); the chief court advisors, Social Knowledge and Ascetic Knowledge, and the bhakti guru, Devotion-to-Śiva. King Life's archrival is King Disease, who oversees an army of disease-soldiers, including Queen Cholera (Vīṣūcī), Crown Prince Pallid (Pāṇḍu), Goiter (Galagaṇḍa), Piles (Arśāṃsi), Vomiting (Chardi), and a host of other unsavory villains.[16]

Act 1 opens with a rather formulaic benediction by the stage manager. The historical and authorial data that the stage manager reveals are noteworthy:

STAGE MANAGER: Listen. Here in the city of Thanjavur country and city people from many places have come together hoping to see the chariot festival of the Great Lord, Śiva. These members of the assembly have become touchstones to discern the gold that is called poetry that moves the heart. They are receptacles of priceless judgment and playgrounds for the Six Philosophical Schools. They are rewards for my austerities, and they have made me eager. My heart wants to honor them here with this play.

ASST. STAGE MANAGER: (Shaking his head.) On what will the play be based?

STAGE MANAGER: I am producing a new play called "The Joy of Life."

ASST. STAGE MANAGER: Who wrote the script?

STAGE MANAGER: Ānandarāyamakhin, the wish-fulfilling tree of the learned poets.[17]

The stage manager's opening remarks make it plainly clear that *The Joy of Life* was written for mass consumption. The play apparently brought people together from all walks of life, from both the country and city, suggesting that the information in the play would be democratically pitched so that people of multiple classes and castes, with dissimilar and perhaps no access to education could benefit from the performance. After several laudatory verses to Ānandarāya and his family, the remainder of Act 1 takes place in the royal fortress of King Life. The narrative opens with a conversation between Social Knowledge and one of his lieutenants, Concentration (Dhāraṇā), who, still wearing the disguise of an ascetic, recounts the details of her undercover work inside King Disease's citadel. She tells Social Knowledge that King Disease is conspiring with his army to annihilate King Life. Concentration's assessment of King Disease's plan and massive military might does not bode well for the future welfare of the king and his allegorical fortress-body, the dual nature of which Ānandarāya simultaneously renders throughout the play with the Sanskrit term *puram*.

The play then shifts back and forth between the two kingdoms of Life and Disease. In Act 2, in the kingdom of Disease, Crown Prince Pallid rallies his troops to discuss the upcoming attack on King Life. King Disease's doorman, Goiter, and some minor lieutenants, Leprosies

(Kuṣṭas), Madness (Unmāda), Ulcers (Vraṇas), Piles (Arśāṃsi), and others, voice their desire to annihilate King Life and his army. The most vocal of the lot are Diarrhea (Atisāra), whose purported expertise is the unstoppable ability to break through a body's defenses, and Abdominal Tumor (Gulma), who boasts that once he gets inside Life's fortress, his malignancy will be swift and sure.

In Acts 3 and 4, the attack on Life's fortress-body by King Disease's army of illnesses is fully under way. Meanwhile, one of King Disease's spies, Ear Root (Karṇamūla), reports that King Life has absconded to an unknown location. In response to King Disease's bombardment, apparently, King Life and his wife, Reason, flee to the sanctum sanctorum of King Life's fortress-body, the Lotus City (Puṇḍarīkapuram). There they meet Devotion-to-Śiva, who teaches King Life that through devotional surrender to the god Śiva he may obtain a therapeutic brew that guarantees supreme longevity. This elixir is an alchemical blend, perhaps suggesting an influence from Siddha medicine, of mercury (*rasa*) and sulfur (*gandhaka*), transubstantiated from the semen (*śukra*) of Śiva and the menstrual blood (*śoṇita*) of Śiva's consort, Śakti. Under the influence of this brew, no disease can harm the king or his fortress-body.

To disrupt King Life's spiritual exercises in the Lotus City, in Act 5, Prince Pallid sends a host of Passions (Envy, Love-and-Hate, Deceit, and Madness) to distract King Life from his meditation. When this fails, Pallid and King Disease fix to target King Life's diet. They send Insalubrity (Apathyā) to lure King Life into developing irregular eating habits in the hope that this will make him surrender to two of King Disease's culinary corporals, Overeating (Atibubhukṣā) and Bulimia (Bhasmakā—literally a "morbid appetite").

Act 6 features a lengthy dialogue between Action (Karma) and Time (Kāla). They recount prior events that took place between King Life and his two advisors, Social Knowledge and Ascetic Knowledge. In the course of their conversation, King Disease and Pallid are said to be taking delight in the fact that King Life is growing apart from his two advisors, whom the king is beginning to regard as proponents of polar opposite agenda for his fortress-body. What is more, King Life had apparently became so smitten with Devotion-to-Śiva (a predilection that does not go unnoticed by his wife, Reason) that he increased the regularity of their meetings in the Lotus City; meanwhile, he moved away from (nearly to the point of ignoring) the counsel of Social Knowledge. During this time of austere religious practice and introspection, King Life relied exclusively on Ascetic Knowledge for direction. The lopsided attention paid to his religious practice had the effect of distracting King Life from the material affairs and immediate dangers that were pressing on his fortress-body, including the difficulties experienced by all of the people–body parts therein. As far as Ascetic Knowledge is concerned, this is as it should be—one solely concerned with release (*mokṣa*) from the cycle of rebirth and matters pertaining to ultimate reality (*brahman*) need not worry about materiality or threats to the body. Ascetic Knowledge in this way personifies the principle of inward-focused action (*nivṛtti*).

Only when there is near-complete ruin around him does King Life begin to take stock of what has happened. After being informed that a legion of diseases has infiltrated his fortress-body, obliterating his once-fortified immuno-defenses, King Life again accepts the counsel of Social Knowledge, who immediately orders that a round of the mercury-sulfur brew earlier handed down from Śiva be prepared. He dispenses it to King Life's entire army. This boosts their immunity against King Disease's attacks, and the healthful troops of King Life ultimately prevail in battle. The action Social Knowledge advises King Life to undertake, contrary to Ascetic Knowledge's navel-gazing ways, symbolizes the necessity of outward-focused action (*pravṛtti*). On the one hand, he advises King Life to fulfill his body dharma, symbolized by the ingestion of the Śaiva elixir, to enhance the body's immuno-defenses; on the other hand, he then urges King Life to accomplish the king's political and martial duties of defending his kingdom.

In Act 7, now that King Disease has been roundly beaten, Social Knowledge advises King Life to revisit Devotion-to-Śiva to continue his religious exercises. King Life goes to her, and in the course of resuming his religious exercises he is visited by Śiva and Śakti. Pleased with Life's devotion, the divine couple grants him pure knowledge of the philosophy of Yoga, the practice of which will enable him to obtain knowledge of absolute reality (*brahman*). Upon attaining this knowledge, King Life is told that he will enjoy a life free of physical pain and disease, and he will experience a sublime congruity between himself and his environment and in his social relationships. This state—freedom from disease and suffering and accordance between self and other—is the very "joy of life" to which Ānandarāya alludes in the title of the play.

Life is joyful, Ānandarāya's play advises, for people who thoroughly understand themselves as embodied entities with important duties to perform in society. To adequately execute these duties, people's bodies must be fit. By virtue of being human, all people are patients in the biophysiologic sense, for human bodies are prone to require medical or some kind of therapeutic care at any given point in a person's lifetime. And while all people are patients because of their embodiment, they are also patients insofar as, once physical health is achieved, people need direction about how to use their bodies in society. Ānandarāya's choice of allegory to capture this dual nature of patienthood was quite ingenious. But we should not only take away the message that, at the end of the day, as human beings we are and always will be patients. *The Joy of Life* is also quite empowering. The play teaches us that even though every person must come to terms with the state of patienthood inherent to being human, according to Ānandarāya's somatic model, each person is also capable of being his or her own physician, a self-healer. Apart from cases in which a person is physically or mentally disabled, there is hardly a more consistently available custodian for the human body than oneself. All the same, in view of King Life's deliberations about his embodiment and dharmic responsibilities, Ānandarāya makes the case that to be one's own physician, especially in times of acute distress, it is perhaps best to be have trustworthy consultants at hand (Social Knowledge first and foremost and, secondarily, Devotion-to-Śiva and Ascetic Knowledge). The lesson to take away from this play is that medicine—based on the ayurvedic classics and with alchemical overtones possibly from Siddha medicine—is designed to create healthy bodies that permit mental clarity and self-knowledge so that, ultimately, people are able to be dharmically productive members of society. Health of the physical body, mind, and society jointly constitute the warp and woof of a joyful life.

The King's Disease and *The Joy of Life*

The story line of *The Joy of Life* develops in the opposite direction of the narrative of the king's disease in the classical ayurvedic sources. Whereas the typical classical medical narrative starts from a cosmic perspective and moves to the world of humanity and human physiology, Ānandarāya's play tells the story of how the structure and functioning of the human body relates outwardly to the world around it, from the micro-physiology of the human body to the macro-physiology of society. The play demonstrates that healthcare is a fine art of adjusting a body's parts and immuno-defenses to support the demands of a person's social relationships and religious duties. Ānandarāya makes the case that King Life has a clear responsibility to care for his body. This is the king's body dharma. His approach to this somatic responsibility is the play's allegorical model for addressing the human patienthood experience. We watch his body undergo afflictions, which interrupt his ability to carry out both routine and complicated tasks. Crucially, we also watch him respond to these somatic setbacks, and see how a person can effectively overcome sickness and restore effective social and religious agency in his or her life.

As was the case in the previous chapter, here too the model of the king is significant. In ancient India many people relied on the king for protection and sustenance, and if the king went down he took many people with him. But the king in Ānandarāya's work should not be read merely as a royal sovereign of subjects and territories, a reading which would inevitably prevent an intimate identification of the festival audience with the play's hero. The allegorical nature of King Life represents a self-sovereign, a person who is simply a king unto himself. Put another way, King Life is an embodied human being. The various predicaments in which he finds himself in *The Joy of Life* collectively formulate an elemental question that arises from being human, a question with which many people at some point in their lives are confronted: How do I superintend my physical body while facing illness, mental unrest, social insecurity, and religious uncertainty? In this way, the basic messages of Ānandarāya's play were sure to resonate with many people.

The subject matter of Ānandarāya's play is diverse and complex, but above all it is about dharma and the ways in which this socio-ethical principle makes sense of the numerous cultural commitments in which people frequently finds themselves enmeshed. The dharma concept is at once descriptive and prescriptive. It operates in this way as both a "model of" and a "model for" reality, not unlike Clifford Geertz's famous explanation of religion as a system of symbols that is both a model of and a model for reality.[18] Ānandarāya crafted the allegory of the king's fortress-body, the puram, to model the complex reality of the human physical condition. Bodies break down. People get sick. At the same time, the fortress-body is a model for somatic improvement. The allegorical duality of the puram highlights the give and take between oneself and one's associates—family, friends, foes—that may contribute to or detract from a person's realization of health. The puram-model illustrates the tenuousness of health, for human embodiment entails a constant negotiation of numerous relationships that have the potential to benefit or handicap one's well-being. Although it might be tempting to become introverted and withdraw into oneself amid social and environmental trials and hostilities, Ānandarāya states in no uncertain terms that introversion and the singular retreat into spiritual activity misses the point of body dharma. That is, the prescription to maintain a commitment to the body that King Life learns in *The Joy of Life* is a vow to support both sides of the allegorical puram—both body and fortress. The fortress is different than but not divorced from the fleshy, skin and bones body with which a person engages the world. It signifies the objects of the body's sense engagements, those things, people, and institutions in the world that a person comes to know, appreciate, cultivate, love, as well as ignore, contest, and battle in life, all of which contribute to a person's overall well-being. That Ānandarāya chose the fortress, a stronghold or fortified place, to dramatize the social side of health and patienthood and the kṣatriya, the warrior-king, as the model for the assignment of reaching a balance between oneself and the external world of others and objects is theatrically arresting. This framework mixes the always-captivating trials and tribulations of the aristocracy, espionage, combat, and religious mysticism with the humor of allegorical unlikelihoods and absurdities. Still, the baseline of the play is the message that the pursuit of joy in life is a battle for health, a struggle that leads to the triumph of either life or death. It is truly disease warfare. And, to be sure, the specter of disease is a somatic fact of life that is neither unlikely nor absurd. It was certainly meaningful for the audience of *The Joy of Life* at Thanjavur's Bṛhadīśvara Temple festival, and it is a lesson that remains significant today.

The use of military metaphors to explain disease pathology and treatment often reflects concerns and anxieties not only about individual bodily health, but also about wider rifts, concerns, and unease in society. Military imagery in *The Joy of Life* links illness and the threat of illness to politics, religion, war, fear, violence, control, and heroism. In so doing, Ānandarāya situates medical discourse amid cultural categories that additionally could have made medical issues more accessible and relevant to a lay audience. This signals, as Deborah Lupton has shown, a utilitarian, state-managed approach to maintaining the health of the body politic:

> While military imagery may overtly connote decisive action and the refusal to "give in" to the disease, at a deeper level of meaning this discourse serves to draw boundaries between Self and Other by representing the body as a nation state which is vulnerable to attacks by foreign invaders, invoking and resolving anxieties to do with xenophobia, invasion, control and contamination.[19]

Ānandarāya's dramatization of the events in a royal body-fortress as a tale of disease warfare makes medical knowledge and healthcare a "culture complex," in the modern sociological sense. His play suggests that a wide-ranging group of cultural traits, including nationalism, defense of the body politic, and religious devotionalism (in this case Śaivism), are dominated and fundamentally supported by the imperative of body dharma. The kṣatriya king, Life, is Ānandarāya's allegorical fulcrum to impart this message. On the health of his body and social productivity all others are sustained. His physical, intellectual, and emotional struggles are every person's struggles, writ large for the stage.

The Joy of Life in effect reiterates what the Sanskrit medical classics established centuries earlier: ayurvedic knowledge offers both empirical and normative information about how to make the human body healthy in order to be able to attend to other duties, or dharmas, in one's lifetime. To maintain a state of physical health, King Life must come to terms with, and ultimately accept, his dharma as a warrior-king. At the same time, he makes a great effort to incorporate bhakti within his dharmic agenda. With the presentation of this balancing act, Ānandarāya is working with a common motif in Sanskrit literature. The question about how best to act in line with one's own dharma evokes the well-known problem in the *Bhagavadgītā*. When the Pāṇḍava warrior Arjuna considers sitting out of the impending battle with his cousins, the Kauravas, the god Kṛṣṇa counsels the wavering warrior. Kṛṣṇa's advice to Arjuna is far from univocal. Yet many commentators on the *Bhagavadgītā* have identified the charge to Arjuna to follow the dharma of his kṣatriya class as basic to Kṛṣṇa's guidance. In one of the poem's most famous passages on dharma, Kṛṣṇa implores Arjuna in this way:

> Look only to your own dharma; do not quiver before it. There is nothing better for a kṣatriya than a dharmic battle. Happy are the kṣatriyas, Arjuna, who have found a battle such as this, the door to heaven laid open. But if you do not take up this dharmic battle, then you will give up your own dharma and fame, and you will gain evil.[20]

King Life's reaction to the attack of King Disease's army in *The Joy of Life* in many ways echoes Arjuna's indecision in the *Bhagavadgītā*. Throughout much of the play, King Life cannot decide if he should be engaged in the world, as a kṣatriya king's dharma necessitates, or withdrawn from the world, leading a life of ascetic contemplation. A central problem for Arjuna in the *Bhagavadgītā* and for King Life in *The Joy of Life* has to do with each individual's understanding of his position and function in the grand scheme of Hindu cosmology.

To figure out his place in the universal scheme of things, King Life weighs the recommendations of his two primary advisors, Social Knowledge (Vijñānaśarman) and Ascetic Knowledge (Jñānaśarman), who separately symbolize, and thus respectively advise King Life to take, the paths of outward-focused action (*pravṛtti*) and inward-focused action (*nivṛtti*). Social Knowledge advises King Life on the "three things" (*trivarga*) every good Hindu should pursue in life: kāma, artha, and dharma. Ascetic Knowledge advises the king about a radically different pursuit, the fourth valid aim of life for Hindus, release (*mokṣa*) from the cycle of saṃsāra. King Life's two advisors press the king towards their respective priorities throughout the play while simultaneously trying to persuade him to reject the advice of the other. Early on, King Life heeds the advice of Ascetic Knowledge, so he devotes the bulk of his energies to transcendental matters of the mind and self. But, as Maria Schetelich has correctly observed, Social Knowledge's rational and grounded way of thinking swiftly becomes vital to King Life's well-being because military and political strategies are needed to keep his body intact against King Disease's assault.[21]

The importance of religion, specifically Hindu dharma and devotional Śaivism, to the maintenance of bodily health in the play cannot be overstated. Religious practice leads King Life to realize perfectly his function on earth as a king, his *rājadharma*, which was of clear importance in the preceding chapter's narrative of King Moon and the king's disease. Here, King Life learns that the dharmic obligations of kings are endless and immense. Ānandarāya has Social Knowledge describe King Life's dharma as involving an array of important outward-looking diplomatic actions:

> By granting favors to old brahmins who have performed difficult religious austerities and by regularly giving gifts to those worthy of donations for their prior devotion, the king protects himself. After establishing his authority over the surface of the earth, the king must govern the whole kingdom. By traversing the path of dharma, the king resolves to protect his subjects thoroughly. In short, every consideration the king has to make is always for the sake of prosperity among his advisors and friends, in matters of the environment, the treasury and housing, and the military.[22]

The description of the king's dharma is in line with the concept of *pravṛtti* that the advisor Social Knowledge represents in the play. Above all, his own safety and bodily well-being, Social Knowledge explains, should be the king's primary interest. Because he is the cynosure of society, his fitness or lack thereof greatly impacts the wellness or illness of his subjects and society. He ensures his own well-being by plying important religious figures in his court with gifts. Such offerings ultimately solidify the religious authorities' loyalty to the king; without it, the king cannot fulfill his dharma as the primary sacrificer in society. Having won the support of the religious leaders, the king should turn his attention to the cultivation of happiness and prosperity (literally "a better tomorrow" [*śvaḥśreyasa*]) among his hirelings and subjects and throughout his territories.

In the end, the actual source of King Life's "disease," that which truly ails him, is the complexity that comes from having to square commitments within one's private life and social life. The view of Social Knowledge is that the highest goal of a king's dharma is the establishment of prosperity in his puram, or body-fortress. King Life cannot create prosperity among the masses until he achieves healthfulness in his own body, however. Whereas Social Knowledge tries to keep King Life grounded and focused on matters of the body-puram so that he can then gainfully support the health of the body politic, the religious practices that King Life learns from his other advisor, Ascetic Knowledge, and his yogic guru, Devotion-to-Śiva, involve therapies to ascertain the nature of his individual self (or ātman), which in turn give his body motivation, focus, and energy to act on behalf of the people within the ambit of his fortress-puram.

Just as Āyurveda gives people knowledge for becoming somatically sound and thus dharmically competent, Devotion-to-Śiva effectively gives King Life the energy to rule, to do his kṣatriya dharma. Without her, he was unsure of himself in the face of King Disease's attack. Because of his relationship to Devotion-to-Śiva, King Life learns about his true self—what he is made of, what he is capable of doing, and what he must do. He also takes on a more balanced attitude and approach to life thanks to her, which favors neither the matters of the spirit nor those of the material world, but instead uses each in the service of the other. He learns a great deal about the importance of religious practice to his kingly dharma, and, like the lesson Arjuna receives in the *Bhagavadgītā*, he learns how the active pursuit of his dharmic obligations may become expressions of his religious devotion to god.

It is not a lesson easily learned, however. In Act 4, not long after King Life exits the Lotus City, he regrets having to stop his devotional worship to Śiva, as well as having to leave his guru, to go and protect his fortress-body. Two friends of Devotion-to-Śiva, Memory

(Smṛti) and Faith (Śraddhā), see the king languishing and encourage Devotion-to-Śiva to visit him. She does. She explains to King Life that although he longs for the spiritual elevation that comes from genuine devotion, the health of the body should be his focus in the present lifetime because it is the support that will enable the fruition of all of his earthly and spiritual goals:

> It has been said that my lord, having remembered me, is regretful and that he has become disappointed with what was done and what is yet to be done. After hearing this, I have come to console you. You should properly adhere to the plan of your minister, Social Knowledge, for the conquest of your enemies. Immediately after that, having conquered all rivals, you will be fully healthy, free from sickness, and rid of disease. And upon returning to me, I will make you the ocean of supreme joy, a knower of ātman and ultimate reality.[23]

Her message to King Life is quite simple and down-to-earth. First things first, she basically tells the king. He must attend to his puram, ridding his body of all illnesses and his fortress of all enemies. The first obligation for King Life is to attend to his body-puram. After that, he should direct his attention to his kṣatriya dharma, namely, his social commitments as a protector of and provider for the subjects of his fortress-puram. Having met these two dharmic commitments—to body and kingdom—King Life may then devote himself to religious meditation and devotion. But the latter cannot occur without the proper attention to the former. Devotion-to-Śiva promises to reward him handsomely for his efforts, making him "the ocean of supreme joy, a knower of ātman and ultimate reality." Appropriate to the genre of allegory, Ānandarāya weaves a great deal of backstory into the somatic lessons King Life continually receives in *The Joy of Life*. In the development of the King Life character, the poet strikes a rather didactic appreciation for and adherence to the institution of dharma apropos this man in a position of power and privilege in Hindu society. He sympathetically acknowledges the blinding attraction of Hindu devotionalism to god, which in King Life's case is deterring him from the dharma of everyday life, and he insists, that without physiologic well-being, everything else falls apart. Because King Disease's army of sicknesses threatens King Life's physical performance, which as we have seen impinges on many others as well, this somatic situation must be attended to before all else. The somatic lesson King Life must learn in this play is a basic lesson. But it is a lesson that becomes complicated as people grow older, learn about the complexities of living a "good" human life, and take on multiple responsibilities that make them dependent on others and others dependent on them.

pravṛtti-nivṛtti / Vijñānaśarman-Jñānaśarman

Underlining the vacillation between his dharmic obligations, his spiritual, or emotional, desire to withdraw into a life of religious austerities in the Lotus City, and his commitment to the welfare of his body is the notion of *vṛtti*—"action," sometimes also translated as "behavior" and "being." In *The Joy of Life,* to address the basic question of how to act in the world, Ānandarāya cleverly presents a fundamental dichotomy of classical Indian thought, that of *pravṛtti* and *nivṛtti,* by allegorizing the two concepts as characters in the play, Vijñānaśarman and Jñānaśarman. These important court advisors sometimes appear as the king's alter egos or imaginary miniatures of the king himself, like the modern comedic angel and devil sitting atop his shoulders urging him to act one way or another. Which advisor represents the angel-conscience and which represents the devil-temptation is not always clearly defined in Ānadarāya's play. In fact, each advisor is portrayed as possessing elements of both conscience and temptation for King Life at various times in the play's seven acts. This suggests that the dictates of Hindu dharma are far from black and white in the course of a person's lived experience, and that there is likely a middle path to be taken that somehow bridges the counsel of both advisors. What is clear, however, is that Ānandarāya crafted the content of the advisors' directions to serve as allegorical tropes for the concepts of *pravṛtti* (Vijñānaśarman-Social Knowledge) and *nivṛtti* (Jñānaśarman-Ascetic Knowledge).

The terms *pravṛtti* and *nivṛtti* are often translated as "activity" and "inactivity," though I would suggest that these translations do not adequately meet the density of meaning implied by the two terms. For example, when the prefixes "pra-" and "ni-" are added to *vṛtti,* the new terms imply the outward expression of action into the world—*pravṛtti* (literally "turning forward")—and a withdrawal or inward turning of action from the world unto oneself—*nivṛtti* (literally "turning back"). They both involve a course of action. To where and whom the action is directed differs, however. But this distinction must be retained. I prefer to translate the two terms as outward-focused action (*pravṛtti*) and inward-focused action (*nivṛtti*). These renderings retain the root meaning of "action" (*vṛtti*) while also pointedly marking the complementarity of the two concepts within a single ideological principle about the human condition. Early in his work on *pravṛtti* and *nivṛtti,* Greg Bailey read these two terms as mutually exclusive and opposing ideologies: *pravṛtti* pertaining to the life station of the householder, *nivṛtti* to the renouncer.[24] Over time he reformulated his position, rightly in my view, to suggest that instead of two polar ideologies, *pravṛtti* and *nivṛtti* in fact represent two "ideal types" that make sense only in relation to one another, and offer "a total world view consisting of two related, if opposite, perceptions of how the world and the person operated."[25]

An imperative of complementarity between *pravṛtti* and *nivṛtti* is evident throughout *The Joy of Life* in the actions of King Life. We observe him alternate between active upkeep and defense of his body-fortress and withdrawal from these engagements to perform religious austerities in the Lotus City. Any propensity the king has to protect the body-fortress reflects the outward-focused path of action (*pravṛtti*) that Social Knowledge (Vijñānaśarman) advises the king is most important in a time of war and potential somatic infirmity. This path is *traivargika.* It guarantees that proper attention is given to the aims of kāma, artha, and dharma. In the case of a king, as we have seen, while these goals apply to himself, he also must do what he can to ensure those under his command and protection also are afforded the opportunity to pursue these three things (*trivarga*). Oppositely, the king's inclination to devote himself to meditation and yogic exercise in the Lotus City mirrors the inward-focused path of action (*nivṛtti*) that Ascetic Knowledge (Jñānaśarman) endorses, ostensibly regardless of the external threat of disease to the puram and the king's dharmic obligations to others. This path, which emphatically requires a more austere and ascetic lifestyle than the path of *pravṛtti* allows, is *apavargika.* A person committed to the path of *nivṛtti* is concerned with the endtime (*apavarga*), and specifically with release of the ātman from the never-ending, cyclic rounds of saṃsāra. In the end, when the curtain falls on the stage production of *The Joy of Life,* the key lesson that Ānandarāya's audience applauds is the life message that when there is equilibrium between the paths of King Life's two advisors, that is, when one strikes a balance between *pravṛtti* and *nivṛtti* in one's life, there is somatic health and social well-being.

The complementarity of the paths of Social Knowledge and Ascetic Knowledge becomes clear in Act 6 of the play, when one of King Life's courtiers, Time (Kāla), recounts for Action (Karma) a conversation between King Life and Higher Knowledge. At this point in the play, King Life is clearly suffering from the attack of King

Disease's army. In the preceding act, we learned that several soldiers of King Disease, such as Leprosy (Kuṣṭha), Envy (Matsara), Goiter (Galagaṇḍa), and others, had managed to diminish Life's vitality while he was not attending to the affairs of his court, but instead was in the Lotus City sitting in meditation and learning yoga. Time tells Action that as soon as Social Knowledge left the king's side to check on his army's defense against the advances of Prince Pallid, Ascetic Knowledge snuck into the king's chambers. Life had not heard from him in a while and was pleased to see him. Life expressed regret for stopping his spiritual exercises in the Lotus City to follow the counsel of Social Knowledge, who had convinced him that his obligation as a king, his *rājadharma*, was to be fully present in his court, especially at a time of war.

Time tells Action that Ascetic Knowledge felt rejected when King Life chose to follow Social Knowledge, so he left the puram. Having learned that King Disease's army was beginning to weaken the king, Ascetic Knowledge decided to try again to convince the king that worldly affairs—throwing one's body into action in the world, à la the path of *pravṛtti*—are treacherous and should be forsaken. Ānandarāya's personification of *nivṛtti* in the character of Ascetic Knowledge and *pravṛtti* in the character of Social Knowledge, and their opposing natures, are nicely articulated in the following verses from Act 6:

> TIME (quoting Ascetic Knowledge): "On account of the miserable advice of Social Knowledge, you have unduly reached this wretched night. O Lord, desirous to be free of my debt to you, I therefore come now with good advice."
>
> ACTION: What happened next?
>
> TIME: The king candidly replied, "Friend, Ascetic Knowledge, after a long time you have appeared. Who else but you can make me better?" And he implored, "Speak that usual good advice of yours!"
>
> ACTION: Yes, and then what happened?
>
> TIME: Then drawing close to the king, Ascetic Knowledge softly explained:
>
> "Everyone knows the body is forever transitory. It is the soil that spouts evil. It is a form that consists of visceral fat,

> marrow, muscle fat,[26] bone, flesh, blood, skin, and hair.[27] In it there is excrement and urine in the viscera and cavities. For discriminating folks [the body] is ultimate suffering and should be rejected. How do those who know what is proper endure here, in this kind of hell?"[28]

For Ascetic Knowledge, human life has a singular aim: release from the suffering that comes from being embodied. He proceeds to tell King Life that complete joy is found only in *brahman*, absolute reality, not in its opposite, the world of humanity. If the king follows the directives of Social Knowledge, Ascetic Knowledge argues that the king will forever be trapped in the transitory, physical world of suffering and incapable of experiencing this joy.

Ascetic Knowledge has to cut short his soliloquy when he hears Social Knowledge reentering the king's chambers. As he sneaks off, Social Knowledge enters the stage, and immediately he can tell the king's attitude has changed. The king suddenly appears utterly at ease about the penetration of King Disease and his soldiers into his fortress-body. In fact, the king appears as if he has relinquished all interest in the affairs of his puram. Social Knowledge rightly suspects that his co-advisor, Ascetic Knowledge, has been speaking with the king. Although he seems uninterested in the condition of his fortress-body, out of respect for his advisor, Life asks Social Knowledge what the front line of the battle looks like. When he learns that the situation looks dire, the king's tenor changes:

> TIME (speaking to Action): Hearing this, the king remembered the words of Ascetic Knowledge. His mind oscillating between the objectives of both advisors, the king resolved to act. His mouth trembling, he said: "Since treacherous diseases naturally arise all around because of Wind and the others (i.e., the doṣas), alas, how can we innately be independent of those tortuous ones while seeking refuge in this fortress (in this body)?"[29]

King Life momentarily struggles with the opposing directives of his two advisors. Does he retreat to the peaceable Lotus City and withdrawal from the world—the path of *nivṛtti*—as Ascetic Knowledge encourages? Or does he attend to his physical well-being, to his body and his subjects, and steadfastly engage the often-harmful world around him—the path of *pravṛtti*—as Social Knowledge urges? It is clear that King Life knows he must act. But the question is how to act.

Time explains to Action that Social Knowledge tried once more to make the case that King Life should not abandon the helm and run off to the Lotus City. The consequences of doing so at this stage would be fatal. Then, after numerous scenes of merely listening to Time's narration, Action asks an important and probing question:

> ACTION: Lord, to what extent is the opposition of Ascetic Knowledge and Social Knowledge becoming harmonized?
>
> TIME: My friend, Ascetic Knowledge thinks about release, while Social Knowledge is concerned with matters of this world. That is their opposition. Why do you ask?[30]

He asks, we later learn, because he suspects that both advisors want the king to flourish. But if Ascetic Knowledge truly desires the well-being of the king, then the withdrawal and detachment he teaches must be tempered in some way by more outward-looking activity, for in Act 5 we saw that all meditation and no leadership makes King Life a sick monarch. Realizing this, King Life again gives the reins of the puram to Social Knowledge, who orders for his army a round of the mercury-sulfur elixir gifted by Śiva earlier in the play. This boosts their immunity, and the reinvigorated troops of King Life persevere.

For Ānandarāya, the *pravṛtti-nivṛtti* dichotomy functions on two basic levels. At the personal level, it defines the balance between body, mind, and self (or ātman) that must be struck by every human being to achieve health. At the interpersonal level, it details an individual's engagements in and disengagements from the pedestrian world and the people who inhabit it. Within the framework of *pravṛtti-nivṛtti*, a host of factors, such as one's duty according to class and life station (*varṇāśramadharma*), determine the extent to which a person may give emphasis to one extreme more than the other on the scale of social engagement and withdrawal. They are not opposing ideologies, but opposite bookends on the continuum of lived human experience.

This message comes across clearly in Act 7, which is the last act of the play. Echoing Kṛṣṇa's instruction to Arjuna in the *Bhagavadgītā*, there Lord Śiva swiftly sums up the two paths of Social Knowledge (*pravṛtti*) and Ascetic Knowledge (*nivṛtti*) and adds an overarching third, the path personified by Devotion-to-Śiva, namely bhakti:

> Since the path of your dear old friend, good-hearted Ascetic Knowledge, celebrated by sages, is difficult for you

> to reach, always honor me. For superior combat, however, Social Knowledge is obliged to be truthful; he alone should constantly develop what is best for you in the world. Always think about Social Knowledge as being no different from Ascetic Knowledge. These two are in your possession, and jointly they bring together enjoyment [in this world] and release [from saṃsāra].[31]

Śiva then adds that the king's body-fortress must be properly maintained first and foremost for the *bhaktimārga*, the path of devotion, to be effective. With this, Ānandarāya allies a medical commitment to the health of the body with religious practice. Medical care is the causative facet of the alliance, for the ability to pursue religious interests ensues only from the achievement of a healthful body. To be sure, Ānandarāya wants his audience to see that the king's heart is with his spiritual guru, Devotion-to-Śiva, in the Lotus City, even if he must prioritize his dharmic obligations. Exactly what lies within the walls of the Lotus City is something of a mystery in this text, however.

Within the Walls of the Lotus City

Does Ānandarāya's Lotus City refer to a historical location? Various references resembling Ānandarāya's Lotus (*puṇḍarīka*) City (*puram*) can be found in Sanskrit literature, although I have not found any direct references to the Lotus City as a seat of Śaiva devotion.[32] Duraiswami Aiyangar's Sanskrit commentary on *The Joy of Life* provides two synonyms: *brahmapuram* ("Brahmā City") and *hṛtpuṇḍarīkam* ("heart lotus"), both of which refer to the site that houses the heart and mind (*manas*) of living beings. Geographical references to the Lotus City place it near Kurukṣetra, the site of the great battle between the Pāṇḍavas and the Kauravas in the *Mahābhārata*. In the *Matsya Purāṇa*, the Lotus City is the name of the "world of the fathers" (*pitṛlokam*), where deceased male ancestors dwell after death and where they receive the benefits of the post-funerary rites performed on their behalf by their sons.[33] In the *Viṣṇu Purāṇa*, we find the phrase "having lotus flowers" (*puṇḍarīkavat*), describing a mountain on one of the terrestrial islands situated around Mount Meru, called Krauñcadvīpa.[34] For King Life, the Lotus City appears to sustain him in a dual-natured way, as Ānandarāya's allegory naturally would have it, on both religious-intellectual and physiologic registers of being.

The Lotus City is a place of intense attraction for King Life. It is more than just a shelter from King Disease's virulent soldiers. Life is drawn to the bhakti guru, Devotion-to-Śiva, who resides there, and his emotional temperament noticeably improves in the play whenever he spends time with her. Moreover, his dedication to Śiva palpably improves his somatic health. His bhakti earns him a fearsome brew that boosts his immunity and ensures lasting physical fitness. Yet, in the end, while the Lotus City is the king's spiritual and religious ganglion, it must be the place to which he withdraws after his rājadharmic responsibilities are met, after, that is, he tends to and defends his body-fortress. Allegorically, the Lotus City is at once a place of sublime devotion accessed with one's mind and a physical site of absolute centrality to the functioning of the body. Carl Cappeller's study of *The Joy of Life* is helpful to make sense of this special location and its multipart meaning. He suggested two possible German translations for the Sanskrit compound *puṇḍarīkapuram*: *Lotusblüte* ("lotus blossom") and *das menschliche Herz* ("the human heart").[35] His second suggestion, *das menschliche Herz*, neatly encapsulates the indispensible and subtle nature of the Lotus City in Ānandarāya's play. King Life retreats into the *puṇḍarīka* of his puram, that auspicious (literally blossoming) place within where he can garner his greatest strength to block the attacking army of King Disease. There he looks deep within himself to learn about the vital stuff of his personality, what motivates him, and possibly determine the most practicable means to deal with the situation in which he finds himself. His Lotus City, at the biological level, is his heart, the physical organ that makes or breaks a person's life. It is also the metaphorical heart of one's character, that from which one's spirit, courage, and self-awareness blossom. The Lotus City is thus a person's raison d'être, literally and figuratively. It is there that King Life realizes his purpose in life, his dharma.

In *The Joy of Life*, the Lotus City is the site of supreme self-awareness and ultimately self-transcendence. There Devotion-to-Śiva educates King Life about the seriousness of somatic attention and medical care, about body dharma. The alchemical complementarity and coming together of mercury and sulfur, allegorized as the adjoining of male and female vitality in the semen and menstrual fluid of Śiva and Śakti, characterizes the dualism of Ānandarāya's message about body dharma. Devotion-to-Śiva teaches the king that the keystone upon which one achieves kāma, artha, and dharma in life and, ultimately, fulfills the quest for release from saṃsāra is physical well-being. But the physical body will not be fully nourished unless one brings the intangible benefits of religious practice and devotional sacrifice to bear upon his or her bodily engagements with the world. Ānandarāya's play is the most extensive and complex medical narrative in Sanskrit literature. Yet, underneath the allegoric ornamentation of the play, the somatic lesson for King Life and Ānandarāya's audience(s) is basically the same as the lessons I discussed in the narratives of fever, miscarriage, and the king's disease: the body is the most important instrument to which all humans have recourse to care for and understand the self, family, and society. Bodily health is the underpinning of the institutions of Hindu dharma and bhakti in *The Joy of Life*. Without it, King Disease defeats King Life. With it, King Life prevails. He is able to protect his puram, provide for his subjects, and return to his religious pursuits with a strong somatic frame. A healthy body repels disease, of course, but the medical novelty of Ānandarāya's play and the tradition of medical narration in Āyurveda is that the health of the body supports the religious life. It is for this reason, in Acts 4–6 of *The Joy of Life*, that King Disease and Prince Pallid are so pleased when King Life grows apart from his advisor Social Knowledge, whose job it is to keep the king focused on the goings-on and well-being of his body-fortress.

Chapter 7

Conclusion

Medical Narratives and the Narrativized Patient

Each of the medical narratives in the preceding chapters in its own way formulates a chain of causation linking self-understanding and action to illness and well-being. From these narratives we learn that a person's grasp of his or her social and religious roles, collectively captured in the notion of dharma, influences the actions that person will make, and the performance of those actions in turn leads to a life marked by either health or illness. There is a mutual referentiality at work in Āyurveda, which suggests, returning to our earlier question in Chapter 2, following A. K. Ramanujan, that indeed there is an ayurvedic way of thinking about bodies and their functions in society. It is a way of thinking about the human condition in which dharma, the body, and health compel and support one another. The particularly unique way of thinking about the body in Āyurveda that I have presented here, seen through the lenses of medical narratives within and about (since *The Joy of Life* is not neatly classified as an ayurvedic text per se) Āyurveda, has not been treated in contemporary scholarship on Indian medical history or literature. A significant portion of the source material in the narratives of Āyurveda, however—such as religious myths and philosophical concepts—have been explored in other Indological venues. People with a deep knowledge of Sanskrit medical literature will no doubt recognize these stories as part of Āyurveda's literary past. But to date no one, from historians of Indian medicine to ayurvedic practitioners, has endeavored to make sense of the function of these narratives within the whole framework of Āyurveda. If they are paid any attention at all, it is invariably a perfunctory nod. Scholars of Indian medicine have routinely explained away these stories as non-medical remnants of a time in India's classical and medieval past that saw authorities within the brahminical institution trying to cast a religious veneer on multiple and sundry knowledge systems, including Āyurveda, so as to increase the purview of their authority in response to rival religious groups, such as Buddhism and Islam, that challenged the old guard of ritual brahminism and its social structure. A major problem with this type of treatment of Āyurveda's narratives, apart from the general lack of historical data to validate it, is that the argument consistently rests on an assumption that the knowledge system we typically identify as India's classical "medicine" should be doggedly empirical. And because most of the Sanskrit sources of Āyurveda present a highly empirical understanding of the human body, incidences of atypical language use, that is, non–chart talk narrative discourse, are difficult to square with the texts and the tradition in which we find them. These stories mark a rather uneasy transition from understanding Āyurveda as a tightly contained empirical system to seeing Āyurveda as a multidimensional narrative that comments on cultural issues far more wide-ranging than the domain of science, especially in the idiom of modern biomedicine, might be imagined to address. As I discussed in Chapter 2, the ayurvedic doṣa-system presents a unique connection between the academic, theory-based foundation of Āyurveda and its narrative discourses, because the doṣas make room for ethical arguments of a more social and environmental, rather than a strictly anatomical, nature. Such an expansive worldview is part and parcel to the ayurvedic way of thinking about the body. It is a multidimensional form of thinking, not only about the human body, which of course is primary to its thought, but also about society and religion. As we have seen, a crucial element of ayurvedic knowledge is information about how best to meet the demands of the Hindu notion of dharma. In fact, ayurvedic thinking presents us with a completely novel interpretation of the dharma concept. It advocates a uniquely somatic obligation—the tradition's body dharma—and it states that the fulfillment of this somatic duty is fundamental to attaining health; at the same time, it states that health in turn is essential to the fulfillment of Hindu dharma.[1] For the commentator Cakrapāṇidatta, care of the body is unequivocally a person's most important duty, precisely because an infirm body is always an ineffective instrument for attending to social and religious responsibilities.[2]

Āyurveda's narratives support the argument that a healthy body is the very foundation of the Hindu institution of dharma, in that the body is the medium with which people can pursue and accomplish duties allied to personal dharmas, such as the performance of sacrifice, as we saw in the narrative of fever; the curtailing of certain social activities and associates, as in the narrative of miscarriage; the fulfillment of one's matrimonial commitments, as explained in the story of the king's disease; and the proper governance of one's subjects and territory, as in Ānandarāya's *The Joy of Life*. Āyurveda's narratives teach us that when people's self-understanding of their dharmic responsibilities are erroneous, their actions are liable to generate scenarios involving other people, gods, and demons that beget bodily illness and dysfunction. Likewise, when one knowingly defies one's dharma, the body suffers. Adapting narrative tales from long-standing mythologies about gods and demons, the compilers and authors of the Sanskrit medical classics attempted to explain what they perceived to be the social and religious dimensions of medicine and somatic health care.

The Sanskrit medical narratives regularly communicate the general lesson that healthy bodies, built up and sustained through physical *and* socioethical preparation, such as diet and exercise *as well as* deeds and religious observances that contribute to personal cultivation, are essential to the refinement of oneself as, for instance, a warrior, an ascetic, a mother, a husband, a student, and so on. The priority of body dharma, then, does not vary from person to person, and in this way it falls within the category of general (*sādhāraṇa*) dharma for all people to heed. Health of the body should be a person's first concern irrespective of class, caste, gender, social position, and down the line through different markers of classification in Hindu society. That said, there are also elements of Āyurveda's body dharma that pertain to the dharmaśāstric category of one's own dharma (*svadharma*), for the realizable features of health that can be achieved in any individual body, as the *Suśrutasaṃhitā* makes plainly clear, differ in every person according to key factors such as age (*vayas*), body constitution (*prakṛti*), digestion (*agni*), season (*ṛtu*), habitation (*deśa*), and the like.[3]

Observed in the narratives of the Sanskrit medical classics and the allegorical machinations of *The Joy of Life*, the body dharma concept interlaces numerous areas of Indian cultural history, and it defies discipline-specific categories of the modern academic sort. The use of narrative in Āyurveda does not detract from the medical sophistication of the "knowledge for long life" (*āyurveda*) expounded in the Sanskrit works attributed to Caraka, Suśruta, Vāgbhaṭa, and others. It enlarges and diversifies it. At the very least, as I have argued in the foregoing chapters, the mere existence of an ayurvedic narrative tradition of telling stories about why healthy people become patients demands that we begin to view Āyurveda, its practitioners, and its literary compilers as active generators of Indian culture. An ayurvedic way of thinking about the body is not an epiphenomenal way of thinking, appropriate only for those who specialize in medical science, although it has been treated as such by historians of Indian history in Western scholarship for decades. Āyurveda's medical narratives show us that health and the knowledge that helps people achieve the somatic condition of healthfulness are part and parcel to the history of the Indian human sciences.

In narrating illness and narrativizing the patient, ayurvedic thinkers resolve to ask, comprehend, and explain, "What makes us human?" This question pervades ayurvedic thinking in the Sanskrit literature. It is always based on the pursuit to know the body and how it works, both as a self-contained physiologic unit and as the instrument of ethically active agents.

Medical Storytelling and Somatic Lessons

Narrative discourses in Āyurveda represent the body as an entity far greater than the sum of its parts. The body appears as a psycho-socio-religious entity in the tradition's medical narratives, which declare when, where, and under which circumstances bodies should act in relation to other bodies and communities of bodies. By homologizing the human and divine worlds in the stories, the compilers of Āyurveda's narratives amplify the perceived significance (within the medical system itself and for patients) of the diseases they present, and they overstate the consequences of either conforming to or transgressing the medical commands their stories relate. Conformity appears to produce the reward of health and disobedience the reprisal of sickness.

It is tempting to read Āyurveda's narrative etiologies of illness with incredulity. Would not the fantastical lives of mythic beings—Dakṣa, Rudra-Śiva, Revatī-Jātahāriṇī, King Moon, King Life, King Disease, and the others—populating the ayurvedic stories examined in this book have been just as unreal and fantastical to people in classical India as they appear to us today? How could stories about divine gods or allegorical characters have any practical value to a medical knowledge system? A critical attitude toward mythic narratives that insists on reading mythology as merely false, as Paul Veyne has noted, "consists of seeing in myth an oral tradition or a historical source that must be criticized."[4] Veyne was primarily concerned about attitudes toward mythology in ancient Greece. But I would suggest that while the ancient Indian, like the ancient Greek, no doubt "puts the gods 'in heaven,' . . . he would have been astounded to see them in the sky."[5] The gods and demons of mythic narratives are figurative models for genuine human conditions; the foibles and delights of the mythic characters represent the concerns of the stories' compilers about the way things were for the people in the societies in which they lived as well as the way they thought they ought to have been—here again, Geertz's typologies of models *of* and *for* human life and how best to live that life are useful for understanding the dual function of the illness narratives in Āyurveda.

The stories of disease and recovery of health in Āyurveda address distinctly medical questions: What is fever? In which ways, for which reasons, and at which times do women experience miscarriages? Does the king's disease affect only kings and rulers? If so, why? If not, why not? But these questions are asked in a manner that might be unexpected to someone accustomed to the non-narrative, often jargonish, discursive style of contemporary ayurvedic practitioners and educators. Āyurveda's narratives deploy metaphorical presentations of culturally fictitious situations amid otherwise rational and clear-cut medical discourses that can rattle the sense of certainty that comes from chart talk and its presumed objectivity. This is because a close reading of Āyurveda's illness narratives, and an exploration of the mythic traditions from which they were culled, shows that the arguments they put forth involve more than biomedical-type anatomy and pathobiology. Behaviors and life decisions that people adopt and by which they choose to live, rather than physiologic pathogens contained in the body, are depicted as bringing about circumstances in people's lives that either engender healthfulness or threaten the integrity of people's bodies and make them ill. Behaviors and decisions are presented as expressions of a person's character and self-awareness of his or her physical, moral, and social identity. To give meaning to a patient's experience of illness, Āyurveda's narratives present events and experiences that explain why certain behaviors and situations can turn healthy people into ailing patients. By giving a narrative arc to patienthood, they also tell a story about how a patient can improve his or her somatic state through the cultivation of both physical body and embodied self.

I have argued that narrative discourses in the Sanskrit medical sources are not exclusive to Āyurveda in Indian history. For example, in the medical stories of fever and the king's disease, the story lines—the destruction of Dakṣa's sacrifice and King's Moon's loss of semen and subsequent wasting—are adaptations of relatively well-known Hindu myths that the compilers of the medical compendia used to accentuate and articulate concerns about the implications of social and religious actions—such as the performance of the sacrifice (*yajña*), sexual licentiousness, and a husband's dharma—on somatic well-being. In the story of miscarriage, the plotline is less common in the history of Sanskrit literature, but the primary characters are important, alternate versions of long-standing mythic figures in both Hindu and Buddhist mythology. Conversely, the story of King Life's battle with King Disease in Ānandarāya's allegorical drama, *The Joy of Life*, is highly unique and, although the story is exceptional, the themes of statecraft and religion framing the medical import of the allegory are decidedly common in Sanskrit literature. The entire play appears to have been a dramatic presentation for laypeople to learn some technical ways in which health and illness are products of the relationships existing among individual human bodies, the state, and religious intuitions.

It is difficult to know how the medical stories of Āyurveda would have been received in classical India, because the Sanskrit sources do not plainly spell out the reasons why a narrative is a better vehicle for patient edification on matters of fever, miscarriage, and the king's disease than non-narrative medical discourse, or chart talk. But because the narratives (or parts of the narratives) were widely known outside the medical context, as I have demonstrated, it is possible, even likely, that the patients of Āyurveda had some familiarity with these stories. Even an informal acquaintance with some of the major components of the narratives could have promoted patient understanding of the social, ethical, and religious bases of the illnesses and, more importantly, ensured patient compliance with the narratives' somatic instructions, the morals of the stories, that convey the prescriptions and proscriptions for patients.

The narratives of Āyurveda are perhaps good examples of what scholars of Indian medical history for more than a century have called the "magico-religious" and "folk" elements of ayurvedic medicine.[6] Many have judged such therapeutics, as Steven Engler has recently argued, to be "either stale Vedic remnants or later Brahmanical impositions that were intended to repress Āyurveda's revolutionary empiricism."[7] There are valid reasons to read the narratives of Āyurveda within a genealogy that has roots in the Vedas. Likewise, as I have shown in Chapters 3 through 6, the narratives of Āyurveda reveal standards and interests that reflect a brahminic influence. I would, however, caution against suggesting that the presence of religious discourse in the medical literature is a mark of the thinking of religious authorities who were intent to repress or in some way discredit the empirical progress of the ayurvedic tradition. This line of thinking anachronistically imposes a modern (usually Western) understanding that the epistemes of science (or medicine) and religion are radically incongruous and incompatible onto the classical and medieval Indian eras. One need not mount a defense of ayurvedic empiricism by attempting to argue away all signs of religious discourse in the Sanskrit medical classics, and only thereby suggest the medicine in the literature has merit. This approach, it seems to me, invariably fails to appreciate the historical significance of Āyurveda in Indian cultural history. To examine the ayurvedic tradition as a whole, the classical texts of which are products of lengthy creations and redactions, not to mention generations of authors and compilers living in cosmopolitan areas, is to acknowledge the profoundly multidimensional episteme of classical Āyurveda, including its straight chart talk of clinical diagnosis and treatment, socioreligious ethicization of narrative discourse, philosophical speculation on karma, saṃsāra and the *trivarga*, and socio-moral-legal statements on Hindu dharma. It is important to situate Āyurveda in Indian history, of course, and to understand the interplay of the different "disciplinary" (in the modern academic sense of the term), as well as perhaps at times competing, dimensions of its reasoning. These dimensions, as I have argued, frequently extend beyond the modern boundaries of science and biomedicine. Āyurveda's knowledge for long life does not appropriately fit within these boundaries. It is unproductive, moreover, to postulate that there ever was a pure "science" of Āyurveda, and on the basis of that postulation pretend to peel away any layers of the tradition that might be judged to be un-scientific for one reason or another. It is not my intention in this book to defend or refute the supposed scientificity of Āyurveda. Instead, I have tried to contextualize three major narrative cycles in ayurvedic history by showing how the components of each cycle have adopted, commented upon, and emended parts of numerous Sanskrit knowledge systems from Indian history. The medical retellings of these stories add new variants to these narrative traditions. By providing the historical trajectories of the medical stories, I hope to have shown how in the medical context the strategic use of narrative discourse, moral language, and stories about certain gods and goddesses can evoke profound and complex inventories of cultural and religious imagery among the hearers of these stories. These hearers comprise an audience that includes physicians, students of medicine, and the sick and somatically unfit (Āyurveda's "diseased ones"). For all of them, the crucial takeaway from these stories is that care and health of the body is contingent upon more than just material medicaments. This literature teaches us that somatic welfare is also achieved through moral, socioethical, and sometimes political means.

The Narrativized Patient

The medical narratives of Āyurveda reflect on and speak to important social and religious dimensions of human life that generally require people to be active, responsible, and productive members of society. Portrayals of the live of patients, especially their actions and decisions, in ayurvedic literature reveal a lot about the tradition's classification of the human being as a patient. The main characters of the illness narratives of fever, miscarriage, and the king's disease are medical patients, so-called "diseased ones." The characterization of patients and patienthood in Āyurveda's narratives differs noticeably from stock portrayals in the medical literature.

To begin, there are some elemental aspects of the representation of the ayurvedic patient commonly found in the medical sources that stand out. Ubiquity and malleability are two defining features of the patient's portrait in the Sanskrit medical sources. Frequently changing from section to section in each source, descriptions of the patient are made to fit the issues of the different medical discussions at hand. Sometimes patients are male, sometimes they are female; occasionally they are old, occasionally they are young; at times they are well built, at other times they are frail. For the most part, where the Sanskrit sources explain diseases of the body, it is understood that the body about which they are talking belongs to a person who is, as is readily seen in the general terms for "patient" like *rogin*, *ātura*, and *vyādhita*, all of which mean "diseased," in some way somatically imperfect. Tellingly, the compilers of the medical sources usually did not use the terms for "patient" in discussions of disease. Instead, they obliquely correlate the object of their inquiries, best described as the "generic patient," with the condition afflicting the patient's body, so that, for example, a patient suffering from a urinary disease (*prameha*) is not called a *rogin*, *ātura*, or *vyādhita* but a *pramehin*, "one who has a urinary disease"; a patient saddled with diarrhea (*atisāra*) is an *atisārin*; a patient with an abdominal tumor (*gulma*) is a *gulmin*; and so on.[8] In this way, the patient becomes the embodiment of disease and a potentially key social vector of illness and infection.

We saw in Chapter 2 that the *Carakasaṃhitā* declares the patient to be one of the four essential elements of Āyurveda. The precise passage from the text reads thusly: "The four pillars [of Āyurveda] are vaidya, medicine, attendant, and patient, [each of whom] is endowed with qualities that should be known as means for the alleviation of disease."[9] Of these four, the patient is the only component tied directly to ill health in the sense that disease occurs in the patient. In the changing representations of the patient's body (as the embodiment of diabetes, of cataracts, of gall stones, et cetera), pathologies are shown to develop, abate, and resurface. The patient is the single sine qua non component of the *Carakasaṃhitā*'s quartet, that thing without which the ayurvedic knowledge system presumably would not have the framework necessary to identify diseases and apply therapies to treat them.

For the compendium of Caraka, the most important qualities of the patient are memory, obedience, fearlessness, and expressiveness.[10] Regarding expressiveness, it is fairly obvious that a physician needs his or her patients to be able to express the nature and history of their diseases to make an accurate diagnosis and apply a proper treatment. During my fieldwork with a family of toxicologists in Kerala, South India, it was common for entire families to accompany patients, not only young children and babies who lacked satisfactory communication skills to explain their situations, but also adults, when visiting an ayurvedic physician. Group accompaniment of a patient was also important in cases in which patients were so injured or distressed that they were unable to communicate their problems on their own. The entourage in effect multiplies the patient's expressiveness by giving perspectival depth to the patient's condition and history (and incidentally underscores the social impact of illness and patienthood in the contemporary ayurvedic context). The second quality, obedience, is vital for the primary reason that a patient must obey the physician's prescriptions and advice for a prognosis and treatment to be effective. Cakrapāṇidatta explains that memory and fearlessness, the first and third qualities in the *Carakasaṃhitā*'s list, are important in a patient because the ability to recall a state of health prior to the onset of illness is useful to recovery; so, too, fearlessness may be advantageous in the face of perhaps painful and troubling conditions that can accompany acute disease and biomechanical dysfunction, not to mention painful treatments. But Cakrapāṇidatta also points out that in some cases, such as insanity and particularly aggressive forms of fever, the absence of memories of past distresses actually may be beneficial to the health of the patient and facilitate healing.[11] The idea of a kind of amnesia or mental suppression of difficult memories evokes the *Carakasaṃhitā*'s prescription of "repression of bad things in one's mind" as an effective means to combat mental afflictions.[12]

Beyond the general fact that patients are humans with bodies that have broken down in some way, the narratives of Āyurveda demonstrate that the tradition's compilers did not solely depict the patient as a mere physical complex of mind, body, and sense organs and a vessel of disease. They also portrayed patients as living and breathing people by attributing to them decision making and experiences, which entail consequences. The decisions and experiences of the patients of the classical medical stories are not just any decisions and experiences, of course. A central function of storytelling in Āyurveda is to articulate events about the lives of people who become saddled with fever because of their religious dissent, about the lives of women who experience miscarriages because of their socially questionable activities, and about the lives of men whose sexual escapades lead to emaciation and an overall burnt-out body. The stories are about ostensibly healthy people who become sick, thus becoming patients, as the result of a series of social and religious actions that create, or are responses to, events that ultimately engender somatic maladies. Āyurveda's narrativized patients are shown to have erred in their behavior in some way, usually for not conforming to the social and religious principles of Hindu dharma as the compilers of the literature envisioned it. The primary dharmic transgressors, that is, the paradigmatic patients, often begin in the stories as well-known gods and goddesses. They are metaphorical exemplars for the human population to observe as models of how not to act. Narrative discourse in Āyurveda thus demands that its audience learn via negativa. The life of the narrativized patient becomes a plot device to demonstrate the ideal ways to somatic health, achieved through an earnest commitment to one's body dharma, which must be inferred to be the opposite of the stories' somatic lessons that link the rise of illness to people's social activities and religious practices.

If the models in the stories are mythic, who then are the human patients, the mortal marks on whom the compilers of the medical narratives set the sights of their analyses? Apart from some general qualities like gender, age, and profession, Āyurveda's illness narratives are about nonspecific, healthy people–cum–ill patients. Moving out of the stasis box of clinical anatomy and into the sphere of social action, the nameless patients of Āyurveda's medical narratives become identifiable as socially active human beings. Patients' bodies and sicknesses in the medical narratives are not mere physical casings and the consequences of a somatic "fault" or "deficiency," the literal meaning of the Sanskrit term doṣa, like we find in the closed-circuit, anatomical bodies that fill most of the "body discussions" (*śārīrasthānas*) in Sanskrit medical literature. Rather, the bodies and ailments of Āyurveda's narrativized patients are integral elements and products of a relational group makeup in which the lives of other human beings, animals, gods and goddesses and the natural world intersect. The patient in Āyurveda's narratives is an embodied self, or a physical body (*śarīra*) with an intangible life force (*jīva*) or ātman motivating it to act in the world.

An important facet of the embodied self emerges in Āyurveda's moments of storytelling—namely, ownership of, and accountability for, the body and all of its social missteps. A person is responsible for taking care of a body and for living life in such a way as to manage, in A. L. Basham's words, "the whole life as to prolong it, and to preserve health and vitality as far as possible."[13] This may be accomplished through a variety of methods, but the tradition's narrative discourses point primarily to actions that are related to socioreligious obligations. The co-occurrence of narrative etiologies of disease alongside medical methods of diagnosis that involve non-narrative and highly analytical thought in the Sanskrit sources suggests that, at least during portions of the tradition's development, physicians were perhaps willing to work with more than one basic explanatory structure. Elsewhere I have described these different structures in terms of the two general body typologies that occur in the classical sources: the anatomico-physical body and the embodied self.[14] The classical compilers ordinarily elaborated the typology of the physical body in aphoristic *kārikā*-style verse common in grammatical and philosophical Sanskrit works (what I have been calling chart talk in this book), whereas to articulate the typology of the embodied self and the life of the patient they employed the prolix discourse of narrative storytelling.

The two body typologies highlight the dual functionality of the patient in Āyurveda's knowledge for long life. On the one hand there is the bodily unit, and on the other hand there is the socially modal patient who uses his or her body as an instrument of socioreligious action and expression. Medical theories in Āyurveda address both areas, corporeal physiology and social agency, with doctrines such as the theory of the three humors (*tridoṣavidyā*) and the standards of right conduct (*sadvṛttam*). From either perspective, they foster the notion that inattention to ayurvedic knowledge can lead to illness. The theory of the three humors is a frequently commented-on aspect of classical and contemporary Āyurveda, which I discussed in Chapter 2. The multidimensional narrative of Āyurveda includes somatic lessons about social and religious behaviors, and these are just as important in medical diagnosis and therapy as humoral theory, to promote, as P. V. Sharma has remarked, "the protection of health in healthy people and the palliation of sickness in patients."[15] For P. V. Sharma, at the base of the entire system of Āyurveda is the "practice of health" (*svasthavṛtta*), which is very much like what I have been calling body dharma, and it unequivocally involves actively and at all times living a healthy life through one's social, religious, and environmental endeavors.[16]

Āyurveda's narratives simultaneously tackle medical, social, and religious aspects of human life. They exemplify a view of lived human life that the compilers of the classical tradition sought to successively present and then knock down. In other words, the medical stories are narratives of disputation. As I have argued above, these stories refer indirectly to the compilers' opinions and concerns about social and religious aspects of life by presenting metaphorical examples of certain reprehensible human behaviors. Reprehensible behaviors in the stories I have looked at here—such as Dakṣa's disrespect and inattention to Rudra at his sacrifice and the excessive lust of King Moon—lead to illness and disease in the bodies of the actors who commit them. The onset of illness and disease, in the end, represents clear disruptions not only to the integrity of the body but also in the lives of the actors who become the medical tradition's patients.

Recalling B. K. Matilal's observation that understanding deepens by knowing what an argument rejects as much as, if not more than, knowing what it supports, I suggest that the compilers of the Sanskrit medical narratives do not directly tell us their views about important social and religious features of human life in classical Hindu society. Rather, they invite us to follow the stories of the narrativized patient along paths of apparent moral indiscretion that they sought to denounce. Why did the medical compilers need to present the wrong answer first? The reason is because the world has always been—in classical India as well as in the present-day United States (and elsewhere)—filled with paths leading to ill fates, and every person at one time or another is liable to walk down those paths to their undesirable ends. If Āyurveda is to fulfill its aim of promoting long life and the practice of health, as Sharma put it, then the recognition that a person's somatic well-being is not restricted to the physiology within the confines of a person's skin is an absolute necessity. To know the complete story of health that is available to every human life, humanity needs to know the complete story of illness. Ayurvedic knowledge, spread out as it is over time and across numerous sources, claims to provide this complex story.

And it is a truly grand narrative. In it, the patient is someone whose life, in one way or another, has become disintegrated. Because of the disintegration of his or her life, the patient plays a modal and physical (rather than a speaking) role as the proponent of various straw-man arguments—easily erected and just as easily knocked down—regarding the connections between actions and somatic health. The construction of the patient in the Sanskrit medical narratives, I propose, serves the role of the ayurvedic variation of the ill-informed opponent that is found in many genres of Indian literature, most notably in philosophical debate, whom a Sanskrit author depicts as the holder of an erroneous or weak "prior argument" (*pūrvapakṣa*) that stands contrary to the author's unimpeachable "subsequent argument" (*uttarapakṣa*) and "established conclusion" (*siddhānta*). Seen in this way, the medical authors collectively assume the role of the medical Siddhāntin, and each patient plays the part of the Pūrvapakṣin. Unlike numerous Sanskrit philosophical discourses, like Patañjali's *Mahābhāṣya* on Kātyāyana's *vārttika*s to Pāṇini's *Aṣṭādhyāyī* and Vātsyāyana's *bhāṣya* on Gotama's *Nyāyasūtra*, which present mock dialogues with opponent interlocutors (Kātyāyana for Patañjali, for instance, or the omnipresent opponents, "some people") who are portrayed as speaking their own positions, the compilers of Āyurveda's medical narratives tackled courses more characteristic of oral histories than philosophical debates.[17] They structure the information to be gathered from the stories of the lives of patients in the forms of "stories that were heard" (*śrutā kathā*) long ago or revealed "in the beginning" (*evāgre*) of time. Recounted by respected medical sages, such as Ātreya Punarvasu in the *Carakasaṃhitā* and Kaśyapa in the *Kāśyapasaṃhitā*, these stories portray the lives of patients through mythic metaphors and anthropological observations to represent philosophies of conduct that the stories' compilers reject as not only wrong but also immoral. The compilers of these stories bolster their sense of ethical normativity by arguing that the behaviors of their narrativized patients lead to somatic impairment, which in turn can disrupt the potential for having a long life and the fulfillment of dharma.

In the narrativization of health and illness as the products of social and religious dimensions of a patient's life, rather than purely effects born of a patient's anatomico-physical body, Āyurveda's illness narratives frame the patient's slide into somatic ruin, experience of patienthood, and potential ascent to health in terms of an ideological conversion. A patient is one who must be transformed from one among the infirm, whose modal states of being in the world are flawed and unproductive, to a healthful person, whose modal states exhibit ethical integrity and physical efficiency. Movement out of patienthood and into a state of physical fitness simultaneously reflects and leads to a resoundingly well-lived life.

Glossary

ārogya — Health or freedom from disease.

artha — Material prosperity; one of the "three things" (*trivarga*).

Arthaśāstra — Name of a Sanskrit book on statecraft from the turn of the Common Era, traditionally attributed to Kauṭilya. Authorship of this book is a point of debate, and scholars also recognize Cāṇakya and Viṣṇugupta as possible authors (or redactors) of the work.

āśaya — Literally meaning "container" or "vessel," this ayurvedic term is commonly translated as bodily organ.

ātman — Often rendered "self," lexically ātman is a reflexive pronoun meaning "myself." In Sanskrit literature ātman is sometimes used to refer to one's physical self, that is, the body. It is perhaps more popularly known, however, as the unchanging element of every person that travels through saṃsāra and is, for some philosophical schools, such as Advaita Vedānta, equal to absolute reality (*brahman*).

āyus — Long life, longevity.

āyurveda — This is a Sanskrit compound meaning "knowledge for long life." As a proper name, Āyurveda refers to the knowledge system originating in the Sanskrit medical classics, which remains a dominant

	medical system in South Asia today and is an increasingly popular "alternative" medicine in other parts of the world as well.
ayurvedic	This is the adjectival form of *āyurveda*. The convention in this book has been not to capitalize, italicize, or place a macron over the *'a'* because the term is not Sanskrit, but an English-language neologism.
Bhela	Name traditionally ascribed to the author of the *Bhelasaṃhitā*.
bhūtavidyā	Demonology; one of the eight branches of ayurvedic medicine.
brahmin	Name of the first of the four Hindu social classes (*varṇas*), typically called the priestly class. Brahmins were throughout much of premodern Indian history the purveyors of Sanskrit knowledge of all sorts, though they are perhaps most often associated with Hindu religious knowledge, practice, and education.
Brāhmaṇa	This proper noun denotes the exegetical or explanatory segments of the Vedas that were developed as commentaries on the mantra portions of the Vedas (e.g., *Ṛgveda*). A Brāhmaṇa may be generally classified as a genre, or text type of Vedic literature (along with *mantra*, *āraṇyaka*, and *sūtra*); it may also specify a Vedic text, in which case the name of the text is affixed with the title "*Brāhmaṇa*"—for example, the *Śatapatha Brāhmaṇa*.
brahminism	Many early scholars of Indian religions used this term to refer to, and thus distinguish, Vedic religion (i.e., the religion of the Vedas and the Upaniṣads) from later, allegedly more corrupt and degenerate forms of modern Hinduism. Along these lines the late nineteenth-century Indologist, Monier Monier-Williams, famous editor of the widely used *Sanskrit-English Dictionary* of 1899, wrote: "The term Hinduism . . . best expresses Brahmanism after it

had degenerated—to wit, that complicated system of polytheistic doctrines and caste-usages which has gradually resulted out of the mixture of Brahmanism and Buddhism, with the non-Aryan creeds of Dravidians and aborigines" (p. 84 in *Hinduism* [London: Society for Promoting Christian Knowledge, 1880]). Thus, early Indologists, such as Monier-Williams and F. Max Müller, to name two of the most well-known scholars, often told the story of the Hindu religion in India as a story of decline or degeneration from an originally pristine, Indo-European, Vedic beginning, with the "decline" into classical and medieval Hinduism (a highly contentious term in its own right) portrayed as an intrusion of non–Indo-European elements (the "creeds of Dravidians and aborigines," as Monier-Williams wrote) into the older Vedic tradition.

Cakrapāṇidatta — Name of the eleventh-century author of the *Āyurvedadīpikā*, a commentary on the *Carakasaṃhitā*, and the *Bhānumatī*, a commentary on the *Suśrutasaṃhitā*.

Caraka — Name traditionally ascribed to the author of the *Carakasaṃhitā*.

cikitsā — Therapeutics, the practice or science of medicine.

Ḍalhaṇa — Name of the twelfth-century author of the *Nibandhasaṃgraha*, a commentary on the *Suśrutasaṃhitā*.

dharma — This word means most basically "duty." Yet it is important to note that dharma is notoriously difficult to translate into English because it carries a variety of meanings in Sanskrit literature, Hinduism, and across Indian history. Etymologically, the term comes from the Sanskrit verb √dhṛ, which means "to hold, bear, support." Hence, and by extension, the idea is that in some sense human behavior done in accordance with dharma is essential to the maintenance of oneself, others, and even cosmological order. In the scheme of the four valid aims of human life in Hinduism (*puruṣārthas*), dharma is typically listed as the third, and it is excelled in importance, if at all, only by the fourth, *mokṣa*, release from the cycle of saṃsāra. The idea that *mokṣa* is in some way an aim superior to the aim of dharma, however, accentuates a potential tension in Hinduism's *puruṣārtha* structure: the idea that the pursuit of *mokṣa* is a valid aim is tantamount to saying that it is a valid dharma, or duty, at least for some people. Yet among the many things renounced by those who genuinely pursue *mokṣa* is the practice and cultivation of dharma. This tension within the *puruṣārtha* structure reveals the complexity and multivalent usage of the dharma concept within Hinduism and Hindu literature. It is often the case that the term dharma carries both a narrow connotation, as in one's own dharma (*svadharma*), which applies to specific religious duties, and a broader connotation, as in so-called general dharma (*sādhāraṇadharma*), which is used in a sociological sense to designate appropriate conduct for all people.

Dharmaśāstra — Sanskrit literature dealing with issues of moral, political, and legal science (e.g., *Manusmṛti*, *Viṣṇusmṛti*, and *Yājñavalkyasmṛti*). The most widely know text from this body of literature among nonspecialists is *The Laws of Manu*.

doṣa — Literally meaning "fault," this term is used in the medical literature to denote one of the three bodily humors: wind (vāta), bile (pitta), and phlegm (kapha, sometimes also known as *śleṣman*).

Dṛḍhabala — Name of the fifth-century redactor of the *Carakasaṃhitā*.

indriya — Faculty of sense, sense organ, bodily power.

Jejjaṭa — (also spelled Jajjaṭa) Name of the seventh-century author of the *Nirantarapadavyākhyā*, a commentary on the *Carakasaṃhitā*, and a partially preserved

	commentary on the *Suśrutasaṃhitā*, the name of which is unknown.
jvara	Fever (sometimes also a generic term for pain).
kāma	Sexual satisfaction; one of the "three things" (*trivarga*).
karman	Act, action, performance. The philosophical concept of causation, ethicization, and rebirth in which a person's every action (*karman*) must have an equal reaction, the effects of which the actor must bear in the present and/or future lifetimes, is typically known as karma (without the final '*n*').
Kaśyapa	Name traditionally ascribed to the author of the *Kāśyapasaṃhitā*.
kaumārabhṛtya	Embryologic-, obstetric-, and pediatric-related medicine; one of the eight branches of ayurvedic medicine.
kāyacikitsā	Internal medicine; one of the eight branches of ayurvedic medicine.
kṣatriya	Name of the second of the four Hindu social classes (*varṇas*), typically called the class of the warrior-kings.
Mahābhārata	This is the longer of the two Sanskrit epics, circa 300 B.C.E to 300 C.E, attributed to the author Vyāsa.
mokṣa	Literally meaning "release," this term is used specifically to refer to the release of the ātman from saṃsāra. The goal of *mokṣa* is traditionally recognized as the fourth valid aim of human life (*puruṣārtha*) in Hinduism.
nidāna	Pathology; the special knowledge needed to determine the cause(s) and nature of disease.
nivṛtti	Inward-focused action.

oṣadhi	Herb or plant, especially a medicinal herb or plant; generic name for a botanical remedy.
pravṛtti	Outward-focused action.
Purāṇas	The Purāṇas are a class of literary texts written in Sanskrit, dating from around the fourth century B.C.E to about the eleventh-century C.E. Generally referred to as the primary mythological texts of the Hindu tradition, in Sanskrit the word *purāṇa* means, adjectivally, "old, ancient, or primeval." As a (neuter) noun, *purāṇa* means "a past event or occurrence," often of a legendary or mythical nature. On the whole, Puraṇic literature celebrates religion, extols kings, sages, and holy men, and is intended for heuristic and devotional purposes.
puruṣārtha	A valid aim of human life in Hinduism, of which there are typically four: kāma, artha, dharma, and *mokṣa*.
rājayakṣman	Literally the "king's disease," this was commonly translated into English in the eighteenth and nineteenth centuries as consumption and tuberculosis.
Rāmāyaṇa	This is the title of the shorter of the two Sanskrit epics, circa 200 B.C.E to 200 C.E., attributed to the author Vālmīki.
rasāyana	Rejuvenation therapy; one of the eight branches of ayurvedic medicine.
rogin	Patient, literally "diseased or sick one."
śālākya	Ear-, nose-, throat-related medicine; one of the eight branches of ayurvedic medicine.
śalya	Surgery; one of the eight branches of ayurvedic medicine.
saṃhitā	The common translation of "compendium" is an extension of the term's adjectival meaning, "conjoined" or "put together." A *saṃhitā* is thus a large,

encyclopedic-type source that brings together copious amounts of knowledge and data in one volume.

śarīra — Body, bodily frame (as in the solid parts of the body).

sthāna — A major section of a compendium (*saṃhitā*).

śūdra — Name of the fourth of the four Hindu social classes (*varṇa*s), typically called the servant class.

Suśruta — Name traditionally ascribed to the author of the *Suśrutasaṃhitā*.

svāsthya — Health; self-reliance.

tridoṣa — The three bodily humors: wind (vāta), bile (pitta), and phlegm (kapha, sometimes also known as *śleṣman*).

Vāgbhaṭa — Name traditionally ascribed to the author of the *Aṣṭāṅgahṛdayasaṃhitā* and the *Aṣṭāṅgasaṃgrahasaṃhitā* (although there is a fair amount of debate about whether or not the same Vāgbhaṭa was associated with both sources, with one or the other source, or with neither of the sources).

vaidya — Physician, one learned in medical matters.

vaiśya — Name of the third of the four Hindu social classes (*varṇa*s), typically called the agriculturalist or merchant class.

vājīkaraṇa — Sexual enhancement, aphrodisiacs, potency therapy; one of the eight branches of ayurvedic medicine.

Vedas — Collective term for the four Vedic corpora: *Ṛgveda*, *Yajurveda*, *Sāmaveda*, and *Atharvaveda*.

vimāna — Measurements; the special knowledge needed to determine the right measurements of such things as a person's doṣic makeup and proper medicines for specific diseases.

viṣacikitsā Also known as *agadatantra*, this is poison treatment or, more generally, toxicology; one of the eight branches of ayurvedic medicine.

yajña Sacrifice.

yuga Cosmic Age; in Hindu cosmological reckoning, there are four *yugas*: Kṛta (or Satya) Yuga, Tretā Yuga, Dvāpara Yuga, and Kali Yuga.

Notes

Notes to Chapter 1

1. Bimal Krishna Matilal, "Scepticism and Mysticism," *Journal of the American Oriental Society*, vol. 105, no. 3 (1985): 480.
2. Rita Charon and Martha Montello, eds., *Stories Matter: The Role of Narrative in Medical Ethics* (New York: Routledge, 2002), xi.
3. Cheryl Mattingly, "In Search of the Good: Narrative Reasoning in Clinical Practice," *Medical Anthropology Quarterly*, 12/3 (1998): 274, 279.
4. KS Kp 2.7–12. There are similar garlic myths in AHS (Ut 49.101) and ASS (Ut 39.111–112). Dominik Wujastyk has translated the mythic history of garlic in the *Bower Manuscript* (*The Roots of Ayurveda: Selections from Sanskrit Medical Writings*, 3rd ed. [London: Penguin Books, 2003], 154–156).
5. Dominik Wujastyk, "The Science of Medicine," in *The Blackwell Companion to Hinduism*, ed. Gavin Flood (Malden, MA: Blackwell Publishing, 2003), 396.
6. Wujastyk, "The Science of Medicine," 396.
7. Rita Charon, *Narrative Medicine: Honoring the Stories of Illness* (New York: Oxford University Press, 2006), vii.
8. Alasdair MacIntyre, *After Virtue: A Study in Moral Virtue* (South Bend: University of Notre Dame Press, 1981), 148–150, 222–225.
9. Mattingly, "In Search of the Good," 290–291.
10. Michael Taussig, "Reification and the Consciousness of the Patient," *Social Science & Medicine*. Part B, Medical Anthropology, vol. 14B, no. 1 (February 1980): 4–5.
11. Dominik Wujastyk, review of *A History of Indian Medical Literature*, by G. Jan Meulenbeld, *Bulletin of the School of Oriental and African Studies*, vol. 67, no. 3 (2004): 404–407. In addition to Meulenbeld's masterful study, *A History of Indian Medical Literature*, 5 vols. (Groningen: E. Forsten, 1999–2002), see also Anthony Cerulli, "Āyurveda," in *Brill's Encyclopedia of Hinduism, Vol. II: Texts, Rituals, Arts, and Concepts*, ed. Knut A. Jacobsen (Leiden: Brill Publications, 2010); Guy Mazars, *A Concise Introduction to Indian Medicine (La Médecine indienne)*, trans. T. K. Gopalan (Delhi: Motilal Banarsidass, 2006); Wujastyk, "The Science of Medicine" and Wujastyk, *Roots of Ayurveda*.

Notes to Chapter 2

1. This list of four components (*śarīra, indriya, manas,* and *ātman*) follows the definition of life (*āyus*) in the *Carakasaṃhitā* (Sū 1.42).

2. CS Vi 8.83; SS Sū 10.3; AHS Sū 1.22. See also P. V. Sharma, *Rogīparīkṣa-vidhi* (Varanasi: Chaukhambha Bharati Academy, 2003), 15–17. The best methods of patient examination (*rogīparīkṣa*) in the classical sources typically involve a combination of physical examination, visual observation, interrogative examination, and inferential reasoning.

3. AHS Sū 2.21; CS Sū 9.3, Vi 8.86. For a concise sketch and discussion of the four pillars of Āyurveda, see Debiprasad Chattopadhyaya, "Tradition of Rationalist Medicine in Ancient India: Case for a Critical Analysis of the *Caraka-saṃhitā*," in *Sanskrit and World Culture: Proceedings of the Fourth World Sanskrit Conference of the International Association of Sanskrit Studies*, ed. Wolfgang Morgenworth (Berlin: Akademie-Verlag, 1986): 575–576.

4. CS Vi 8.94: āturas tu khalu kāryadeśa. The commentator Ḍalhaṇa draws the parallel between the body of the patient (*āturaśarīraṃ*) and the earth (*bhūmi*—commentary on SS Sū 35.39–40).

5. I use the common terms "biomedicine" and "allopathy" (and their related adjectives, biomedical and allopathic) for the sake of convenience throughout this book. In personal conversations and in print, Dominik Wujastyk ("Regulation of Āyurveda in Great Britain in the Twenty-First Century," *Asian Medicine: Tradition and Modernity*, vol. 1, no. 1, 2005) has suggested the use of the acronyms MEM ("Modern Establishment Medicine") and CAM ("Complementary and Alternative Medicine") as a way to differentiate so-called Western biomedicine (founded on the medical treatises of Hippocrates and Galen) from all other medical traditions. According to Wujastyk's terms, Āyurveda belongs to CAM. Although I am sympathetic with the effort to avoid the often distortive baggage that accompanies the equation of biomedicine with such categories as the West and science, which imply that medical systems in non-Western societies are fundamentally different from medical systems in Europe and North America insofar as they do not tackle rational or "scientific" issues such as biology and anatomy, I am inclined to avoid using an acronymic designation for Āyurveda in favor of using its self-designation as "knowledge for long life," the literal meaning of the Sanskrit term *āyurveda*. Moreover, as it turns out, in my experience the most common way for ayurvedic practitioners to refer to their colleagues trained in the system of medicine derived from ancient and classical Greco-Roman medicine is to use the terms "allopathy" and "biomedicine." Because I am not interested in theorizing the concepts and linguistic implications of these labels in this book, I defer to the texts and practitioners of Āyurveda on this matter and adopt the terminologies they employ.

6. Michel Foucault, *The Birth of the Clinic: An Archaeology of Medical Perception*, trans. A. M. Sheridan Smith (New York: Vintage Books, 1973), 59.

7. Foucault, *The Birth of the Clinic*, 59–62.

8. Deborah Lupton, *Medicine as Culture: Illness, Disease and the Body in Western Societies*, 2nd ed. (London: Sage Publications, 2004), 84–91.

9. CS Sū 30.27; SS Sū 1.13.

10. On the overlap and potential influences of Buddhism on Āyurveda, see Kenneth G. Zyzk, *Asceticism and Healing in Ancient India: Medicine in the Buddhist Monastery* (Oxford: Oxford University Press, 1991).

11. Ayurvedic colleges in India today teach "the science of the body's arrangement" (*śarīraracana-vijñāna*), which is generally referred to as "anatomy" in English.

12. CS Śā 7.1–4; SS Śā 4.4, 5.6; BS Śā 7.1.

13. CS Śā 7.6; SS Śā 5.18; BS Śā 7.2; KS Śā 2.

14. CS Śā 7.14; SS Śā 5.29; AHS Śā 3.17; ASS Śā 5.49; BS Sū 26.17, 28–29 and Ci 13.18.

15. CS Śā 7.14; SS Śā 5.6, 6.3; AHS Śā 3.39–40.1; ASS Śā 6.28; KS Śā 2.

16. Mazars, *A Concise Introduction to Indian Medicine*, 84–85.

17. Kenneth G. Zyzk, "The Evolution of Anatomical Knowledge in Ancient India, with Special Reference to Cross-Cultural Influences," *Journal of the American Oriental Society*, vol. 106, no. 4 (Oct–Dec 1986): 687–691, 697.

18. CS Ci 3.4, 12.

19. Commentary on CS Ci 3.5–10 ("tumor," *arbuda*, "adherence to untruths," *atattvābhiniveśa*, "partial blindness," *timira*).

20. AHS Sū 1.20–21.

21. CS Sū 11.45.

22. SS Sū 1.23–26.

23. Dominik Wujastyk, "Interpréter L' Image du Corps Humain dans L' Inde Pré-Moderne," in *Images du corps dans le monde hindou*, ed. Véronique Bouillier and Gilles Tarabout (Paris: CNRS-Éditions 2002): 77–78, 80.

24. Francis Zimmermann, "Remarks on the Conception of the Body in Ayurvedic Medicine," *South Asian Digest of Regional Writing*, vol. 8 (1979): 15–16.

25. KS Kp 6.30–31.

26. CS Sū 10.9–10; AHS Sū 30–35.

27. CS Sū 10.7–8.

28. Sharma, *Rogī-parīkṣa-vidhi*, 383; Wujastyk, *Roots of Ayurveda*, 13.

29. CS Sū 11.54—*daivavyapāśrayāuṣadha*, *yuktivyapāśrayāuṣadha*, and *sattvāvajayāuṣadha*, respectively (cf. ASS Sū 1.48–49, 12.5; cf. AHS Sū 1.25–26). And yet there is no conventional line of demarcation—no veritable ayurvedic *lakṣmaṇarekhā*—occluding overlap or shared procedures among these three methods of treatment. As Arion Roşu has noted, "L'âyurveda, qui est une medecine rationnelle dans son enseignement fondamental, comporte aussi, bien que rarement, des pratiques magico-religieuses" ("Etudes âyurvédiques III: Les carrés magiques dans la médecine indienne," in *Studies on Indian Medical History*, ed. G. Jan Meulenbeld and Dominik Wujastyk, 1987 [reprint, Delhi: Motilal Banarsidass 2001], 103).

30. KS Ind 1.3–4.

31. CS Vi 8.87.

32. Commentary on CS Sū 11.54.

33. My ideas about the doṣas presented here are more fully elaborated in my essay for the *Brill Encyclopedia of Hinduism*, "Āyurveda," 274–275.

34. Wujastyk, *Roots of Ayurveda*, xvii.

35. Harmut Scharfe, "The Doctrine of the Three Humors in Traditional Indian Medicine and the Alleged Antiquity of Tamil Siddha Medicine," *Journal of the American Oriental Society*, vol. 119, no. 4 (Oct.–Dec. 1999); Zysk, *Asceticism and Healing*, 29.

36. Some scholars have suggested that there are reasons within Āyurveda itself to translate the term doṣa as "humor," as I do here, for the same reason that the Greeks used the term "humor" (χυμός, literally "juice" or "sap") in the Hippocratic tradition. In ancient and medieval European medical history, there were thought to be four cardinal humors in the human body: blood, phlegm, choler (or yellow bile), and black choler (or melancholy). The relative proportions and locations of the humors were thought to determine a person's temperament, mental faculties, and overall bodily health. On this, see Francis Zimmermann, "Terminological Problems in the Process of Editing and Translating Sanskrit Medical Texts," in *Approaches to Traditional Chinese Medical Literature*, ed. Paul Unschuld (Dordrecht: Kluwer Academic, 1989), 127–130, 177–187; Jean Filliozat, *The Classical Doctrine of Indian Medicine: Its Origins and Greek Parallels*, trans. Dev Raj Chanana (Delhi: Munshiram Manoharlal, 1964), 28–31, 197ff.

37. CS Śā 5.3.

38. Gerald Larson, "Āyurveda and the Hindu Philosophical Systems," *Philosophy East and West*, vol. 37, no. 3 (July 1987): 245–259; Antonella Comba, "Carakasaṃhitā, Śārīrasthāna I and Vaiśeṣika Philosophy," in *Studies on Indian Medical History* (1987), ed. G. Jan Meulenbeld and Dominik Wujastyk (reprint, Delhi: Motilal Banarsidass, 2001).

39. For an excellent historical survey of the five great elements in Sanskrit literature and Indian history, see Karin Preisendanz, "Mahābhūtas," in *Brill's Encyclopedia, Vol. II: Texts, Rituals, Arts, and Concepts*, ed. Knut A. Jacobsen (Leiden: Brill Publications, 2010), 806–818. Although this essay does not address classical Āyurveda directly, Preisendanz provides detailed accounts of classical Sāṃkhya, Buddhism, and Vaiśeṣika, among other traditions, which in many ways illustrate coeval (if not shared) developments in classical ayurvedic thinking on the material makeup of the body and cosmos.

40. CS Śā 5.5.

41. Lakshmi Kapani, "Note on the Garbha-Upaniṣad" and "Upaniṣad of the Embryo," in *Fragments for a History of the Human Body*, ed. Michel Feher, Ramona Naddaff, and Nadia Tazi (New York: Zone Books, 1989), 176–179, 180–196.

42. Larson provides the Sanskrit text and a translation of Īśvarakṛṣṇa's *Sāṃkhyakārikā* in *Classical Sāṃkhya*, 5th ed. (Delhi: Motilal Banarsidass, 2005), Appendix B: passim and 256, fn. 3.

43. For example, see Larson, *Classical Sāṃkhya*, 88, 95–103, 167.

44. Tracy Pintchman, *The Rise of the Goddess in the Hindu Tradition* (Albany: State University of New York Press, 1994), 86.

45. Gerald Larson, "Karma as a 'Sociology of Knowledge' or 'Social Psychology' of Process / Praxis," in *Karma and Rebirth in Classical Indian Traditions*, 1980, ed. Wendy Doniger O'Flaherty (reprint, Delhi: Motilal Banarsidass, 1983), 307–312.

46. Larson, "Āyurveda and the Hindu Philosophical Systems," 258, fn. 7.

47. Zimmermann, *The Jungle and the Aroma of Meats*, 190.

48. McKim Marriott, "Hindu Transactions: Diversity without Dualism," in *Transaction and Meaning: Directions in the Anthropology of Exchange and Symbolic Behavior*, ed. B. Kapferer (Philadelphia: Institute for the Study of Human Issues, 1976), 110–111.

49. Zimmermann, "Ṛtu-Sātmya: The Seasonal Cycle and the Principle of Appropriateness," trans. M. Marriott and J. Leavitt, *Social Science & Medicine*, Part B, Medical Anthropology, vol. 14B, no. 2 (May 1980): 101. Zimmermann has dealt with ayurvedic cosmology and the openness and boundedness of the body in Āyurveda elsewhere, too (e.g., *The Jungle and the Aroma of Meats*, 218–223 and "'May Godly Clouds Rain For You!,': Metaphors of Well-Being in Sanskrit," *Studia Asiatica*, V [2004]: 7–11).

50. David Gordon White, *The Alchemical Body: Siddha Traditions in Medieval India* (Chicago: University of Chicago Press, 1996), 15–23, 218–262.

51. Zimmermann, *The Jungle and the Aroma of Meats*, 190.

52. CS Sū 1.43: tasy' āyuṣaḥ puṇyatamo vedo vedavidāṃ mataḥ / vakṣyate yan manuṣyāṇāṃ lokayor ubhayor hitam.

53. Dominik Wujastyk, "Medicine and Dharma," *Journal of Indian Philosophy*, vol. 32 (2004): 837.

54. E.g., CS Sū 11.25, 11.47, 30.24; CS Si 12.35; AHS Sū 2.30. Occasionally, as we will see in the next chapter, release from the cycle of rebirth (*mokṣa*) is also promoted as a valid life goal in ayurvedic literature, bringing the total number of life goals to four and thus matching Hinduism's "aims of humankind," *puruṣārthas*.

55. On the notion of "personal cultivation" in Āyurveda, see Surendranath Dasgupta, *A History of Indian Philosophy*, vol. II, 5th ed. (London: Cambridge University Press, 1968), 405ff; Anthony Cerulli and Brahmadathan U. M. T., "Know Thy Body, Know Thyself: Decoding Knowledge of the Ātman in Sanskrit Medical Literature," *Journal of Indian Medicine*, vol. 2, no. 3 (2009): 101–107; and Anthony Cerulli, "Religio-Medical Perspectives on the Body, Self, and Embodiment in Āyurveda," in *Refiguring the Body: Embodiment in South Asian Religions*, ed. Barbara Holdrege and Karen Pechilis (Albany: State University of New York Press, forthcoming).

56. CS Ci 1.4.61: na hi jīvitadānāddhi dānamanyadviśiṣyate.

57. A. F. Rudolf Hoernle, *Studies in the Medicine of Ancient India: Part I, Osteology or the Bones of the Human Body* (Oxford: Clarendon Press, 1907); Zysk, "The Evolution of Anatomical Knowledge"; Tsutomu Yamashita,

"Śārīrasthāna of the Āyurveda—A Comparative Study," *Studies in the History of Indian Thought,* vol. 7 (1995).

58. It is not until much later, around the late eighteenth century, that we find medical manuscripts in South Asia with medical illustrations (Wujastyk, "Interpréter L' Image du Corps Humain," 78; *Roots of Ayurveda,* 70).

59. Wujastyk, *Roots of Ayurveda,* xvi; Kanjiv Lochan, *Medicines of Early India* (Varanasi: Chaukhambha Sanskrit Bhawan, 2003), 70–71.

60. Yamashita, "Śārīrasthāna of the Āyurveda," 1.

61. Steven Engler, "'Science' vs. 'Religion' in Classical Ayurveda," *Numen,* vol. 50 (2003): 445.

62. Harmut Scharfe, "The Doctrine of the Three Humors," 612–614; Wujastyk, *Roots of Ayurveda,* 14.

63. Wujastyk, *Roots of Ayurveda,* xvi.

64. A. L. Basham, "The Practice of Medicine in Ancient and Medieval India," in *Asian Medical Systems: A Comparative Study,* ed. Charles Leslie (Berkeley: University of California Press, 1976), 21; Wujastyk, *Roots of Ayurveda,* 3.

65. Zysk, *Medicine in the Veda: Religious Healing in the Veda,* 1985 (reprint, Delhi: Motilal Banarsidass, 1996), 1.

66. SS Sū 1.6; CS Sū 30.20–21; see also Zysk, *Medicine in the Veda,* 25–26.

67. Zysk, *Medicine in the Veda,* 10.

68. Wujastyk, *Roots of Ayurveda,* 3–5, 63–64. See also Meulenbeld, *HIML,* IA: 350–352 and Zysk, *Asceticism and Healing,* 13–17, 21–33.

69. For more information on the history of the medical literature and the contemporary curricula of Government Ayurvedic Colleges in India, see Cerulli, "Āyurveda," 267–273, 277–279.

70. Wujastyk, *Roots of Ayurveda,* 3.

71. Engler, "'Science' vs. 'Religion,'" 446; P. V. Sharma, *Āyurved kā Vaijñānik Itihās,* 7th ed., Jaikrishnadas Ayurveda Series, no. 1 (Benares: Chowkhamba Orientalia, 2003), 113–119; Julius Jolly, *Indian Medicine,* trans. C. G. Kashikar, 3rd ed. (Delhi: Munshiram Manoharlal, 1994), 13–14.

72. A table of contents and the names of the 120 chapters are listed at CS Sū 30.33–35.

73. Meulenbeld, *HIML,* IA, 191–194. P. V. Sharma places Jejjaṭa's commentary on the *Carakasaṃhitā* in the beginning of the ninth century C.E. (*Āyurved kā Vaijñānik Itihās,* 226).

74. Meulenbeld, *HIML,* IA: 182–185; Dasgupta, *A History of Indian Philosophy,* II: 431.

75. Wujastyk, *Roots of Ayurveda,* 3.

76. For example, see Larson, *Classical Sāṃkhya,* 88, 95–103, 167.

77. Lochan, *Medicines of Early India,* 77–81; Frances Wood, *The Silk Road: Two Thousand Years in the Heart of Asia* (Berkeley: University of California Press, 2002), 13, 36–41; Elizabeth Ten Grotenhuis, *Along the Silk Road* (Washington, DC: Arthur M. Sackler Gallery, Smithsonian Institute, 2002), 15–23; Romila Thapar, *Early India: From the Origins to AD 1300* (London: Penguin Press, 2002), 237–244.

78. Sheldon Pollock, *The Language of the Gods in the World of Men: Sanskrit, Culture, and Power in Premodern India*, 2006 (reprint, Delhi: Permanent Black, 2007), 486.

79. Zysk, *Asceticism and Healing*, 46–47.

80. Thapar, *Early India*, 239.

81. Ci 30.289–90; Si 12.37–40. It is difficult to determine with certainty which chapters in the CS Cikitsāsthāna might have been added by Dṛḍhabala, because, as Philipp Maas has suggested, "the sequence of chapters varies in different versions of the Cikitsāsthāna—as well as in different versions of the 'table of contents' towards the end of the Sūtrasthāna" ("On What Became of the *Carakasaṃhitā* After Dṛḍhabala's Revision," *Journal of Indian Medicine*, vol. 3 [2010]: 4).

82. Meulenbeld, *HIML*, IA: 105–109.

83. Commentary on CS Sū 1.4, translation in Maas, "On What Became of the *Carakasaṃhitā*," 3, fn. 4.

84. CS Sū 1.3–5; see also Ci 1.4.3.

85. SS Sū 1.7, 18; 3.45.

86. Meulenbeld, *HIML*, IA: 333–342. See also Wujastyk, *Roots of Ayurveda*, 63–64.

87. MBh Anuśāsana Parvan 4.54–55.

88. GP 149.43; AP 279, 292.

89. K. R. Srikanta Murthy, "Suśruta," in *History of Medicine in India: From Antiquity to 1000 A.D.*, ed. P. V. Sharma (New Delhi: Indian National Science Academy 1992), 197–198.

90. *HIML*, IA: 358; SS Sū 1.21.

91. *HIML*, IA: 362–363; SS Sū 1.3.

92. A table of contents with the names of the various chapters is listed at SS Sū 3.

93. Meulenbeld argues that the name of Jejjaṭa's commentary is unknown (*HIML*, IA: 192, 285). Dasgupta noted, however, "Jejjaṭa's commentary passed by the name of *Bṛhallaghupañjikā*" (*A History of Indian Philosophy*, II: 428).

94. On Cakrapāṇidatta's *Bhānumatī*, see Meulenbeld, *HIML*, IA: 374–375; Srikanta Murthy, "Suśruta," 201; Dasgupta, *A History of Indian Philosophy*, II: 427–428. On Ḍalhaṇa's *Nibandhasaṃgraha*, see Meulenbeld, *HIML*, IA: 376–379; Srikanta Murthy, "Suśruta," 201; Dasgupta, *A History of Indian Philosophy* II: 427.

95. Meulenbeld has adduced fifty-three different medical treatises ascribed to someone named Nāgārjuna. Of course, not all of them are from the classical period. For an overview of the long-standing debate about who the redactor Nāgārjuna might have been, see Meulenbeld, *HIML*, IA: 338–341, 363–368 and Dasgupta, *A History of Indian Philosophy*, II: 424–427.

96. A. K. Ramanujan, "Is There an Indian Way of Thinking?," in *India through Hindu Categories*, ed. McKim Marriott (New Delhi: Sage Publications, 1990), 47.

97. Zimmermann, "Remarks on the Conception of the Body," 11 on the Conception of the Body in Ayurvedic Medicine," *South Asian Digest of Regional Writing*, vol. 8 (1979): 11.

98. The present discussion of Francis Zimmermann's remarks on anatomy, and the lack of anatomical thinking in Āyurveda, is by no means meant to be exhaustive apropos the twinned context-sensitive and context-free thinking in Āyurveda. His 1979 article, "Remarks on the Conception of Body in Ayurvedic Medicine," effectively initiated what would develop into highly creative and influential studies in subsequent years that further refine and articulate the structure of (a)contextual thinking in homological presentations of the body in ayurvedic literature. The article "Ṛtu-Sātmya" and the book *The Jungle and the Aroma of Meats* are classic examples of Zimmermann's work to this end.

99. Ramanujan, "Is There an Indian Way of Thinking?," 52.

100. Ramanujan, "Is There an Indian Way of Thinking?," 54.

101. Ramanujan, "Is There an Indian Way of Thinking?," 55. Ramanujan brilliantly illustrates the two sides of Indian thinking in this now-classic essay. He concludes, however, that even "the 'modern,' the context-free, becomes one more context," mischievously adding, "though it is not easy to contain" (p. 57).

102. Zimmermann, "Remarks on the Conception of the Body," 15; emphasis in the original.

103. ṚV 1.162.16–20.

104. Hoernle, *Studies in the Medicine of Ancient India*, passim; Zysk, "Evolution of Anatomical Knowledge," 687–705; Heinrich Zimmer, *Hindu Medicine*, 1948 (reprint, New York: Arno Press, 1979), 169–177; Basham, "The Practice of Medicine," 27–29. Of the four scholars mentioned, Hoernle and Zysk adduce the most comprehensive and careful accounts of so-called anatomical knowledge in India.

105. Zimmermann, "Remarks on the Conception of the Body," 11.

106. Zimmermann, "Remarks on the Conception of the Body," 10.

107. CS Sū 1.49–52.

108. Many Western scholars have assumed that it does: Monier Monier-Williams, ed., *Sanskrit-English Dictionary: Etymologically and Philologically Arranged with Special Reference to Cognate Indo-European Languages*, 1899 (reprint, Delhi: Motilal Banarsidass, 1997), 122, s.v. "asthi"; Edward Delavan Perry, *A Sanskrit Primer Based on the Leitfaden für den Elementar-Cursus des Sanskrit of Professor Georg Bühler of Vienna* (Boston: Ginn and Company, 1885), 106, s.v. "asthan"; Charles Rockwell Lanman, *A Sanskrit Reader, with Vocabulary and Notes*, Parts I and II (London: Trübner & Co., Ludgate Hill, 1884), 123, s.v. "ásthi"; William Dwight Whitney, *A Sanskrit Grammar: Including Both the Classical Language and Older Dialects, of Veda and Brahmana*, 3rd ed. (Leipzig: Breitkopf and Härtel; Boston: Ginn & Company, 1896), 122, 431; 522, s.v. "asthán, ásthi."

109. Ramanujan, "Is There an Indian Way of Thinking?," 54.

Notes to Chapter 3

1. CS Ci 3.4, 12. Similarly, the *Bhelasaṃhitā* states that "fever is proclaimed the king of all diseases" (rogānīkasya sarvasya jvaro rājā prakīrtita—Ci 1.5).

2. The *Carakasaṃhitā* uses variable terminology to describe the life junctures of birth and death. For example, at Ci 3.5 we find *pralayodaye*, "at the time of dissolution and becoming visible" (i.e., death and birth), while at Ci 3.26 the text reads *janmādau nidhane*, "at the start of birth and at death."

3. CS Ci 3.31: jvarapratyātmikaṃ liṅgaṃ saṃtāpo dehamānasaḥ / jvareṇ' āviśatā bhūtaṃ na hi kiñcin na tapyate. In his *Āyurvedadīpikā*, Cakrapāṇidatta glosses *saṃtāpaḥ* simply as "pain" (*pīḍā*). In the cases of bodily and mental fever, he takes *saṃtāpaḥ* to denote, respectively, rising temperature and distaste.

4. CS 3.14–25.

5. The classical sources generally differentiate "actions" (*karmans*) that were done in past lives (*daiva*) from those that are done in the present life (*puruṣakāra*), the latter of which is the focus here (e.g., CS Vi 3.29–30; Śā 1.116–117). The classical sources also taxonomize diseases as those that arise from problems among the bodily humors (*doṣaja*) and those that arise from actions (*karmaja*—e.g., SS Ut 40.163–165; AHS Sū 12.57–59).

6. There is much debate in ayurvedic literature about the prioritization of these four "aims of humankind" (*puruṣārthas*). The first three, commonly called the *trivarga* in the Sanskrit medical sources—kāma, artha, and dharma—are generally accepted across the literature. The fourth goal, *mokṣa*, "release" from the cycle of rebirth, receives varying degrees of acceptance as a valid human pursuit in the medical literature (e.g., CS Sū 1.15, 12.13).

7. There is a lot of information on fever in Bhāvamiśra's *Bhāvaprakāśa* (Madhyakhaṇḍa, Jvarādhikāraḥ). The *Bhāvaprakāśa* is in large part a commentary, a series of clarifications (*prakāśas*), on the important medical compendia compiled prior to Bhāvamiśra's life (sixteenth century C.E.), and I do not discuss Bhāvamiśra's account of fever (Jvarādhikāraḥ) here. That said, it is worthwhile to mention that Bhāvamiśra's work has been and is still today important to Āyurveda. Bhāvamiśra advanced ayurvedic medicine in a number of important ways: the *Bhāvaprakaśa* was the first Sanskrit medical work to mention drugs indigenous to countries outside India; it was the first to describe and recommend a treatment for syphilis (*phiraṅgaroga*); it formulated contraceptives; and it gave the first accurate account of lathyrism, a type of leg paralysis (Sharma, *Āyurved kā Vaijñānik Itihās*, 206, 211–212, 254; Wujastyk, *Roots of Ayurveda*, xxvii–xxviii).

8. Manu 9.128; BVP Pūrvakhaṇḍa, 6.

9. MBh Ādiparvan 7.114, Āraṇyakaparvan 35.160. In the story of the creation of the universe in the *Kūrma Purāṇa*, Dakṣa, one of the primeval seers, springs to life not from Brahmā's thoughts but from his breath (KP 1.7.30–58).

10. In the ṚV, the Ādityas range in number from six (2.27.1), seven (9.114), or eight (10.72.8); see also ŚB 2.6.3.8, and MBh Ādiparvan 121. Aditi is called Dakṣa's daughter at ṚV 10.72.4–5.

11. Wendy Doniger O'Flaherty, *Hindu Myths: A Sourcebook Translated from the Sanskrit* (London: Penguin Books, 1975), 323–325, 341.

12. W. J. Wilkins, *Hindu Mythology, Vedic and Purāṇic*, 1882 (reprint, Varanasi: Indological Book House, 1972), 372–380; Wendy Doniger O'Flaherty, *Śiva: The Erotic Ascetic* (Oxford: Oxford University Press, 1973), 128.

13. Regarding the patron deity of health and medicinal herbs, see ṚV 1.43.4; 1.114.5; 2.33.2, 4, 12–13; 5.42.11; 6.74.3; 7.46.3.

14. Kenneth G. Zysk, "Fever in Vedic India," *Journal of the American Oriental Society*, vol. 103, no. 3 (July–September 1983): 617–618.

15. YV 3.61. At YV 3.60 Rudra is called Tryambaka ("Three Eyed One"), a name regularly applied to Śiva.

16. O'Flaherty, *Śiva: The Erotic Ascetic*, 83.

17. The educational scenario presented here, in which a teacher (*guru*) expounds a lesson to a student (*śiṣya*), who occasionally interrupts to ask questions, reflects the traditional method and setup of ayurvedic education known as *gurukula*, literally "family of the teacher." In the narratives of the Sanskrit medical classics, the portrayal of the guru-śiṣya arrangement is ubiquitous.

18. This formidable child born of the fire of Rudra's anger is called Vīrabhadra in some Purāṇic versions of "Dakṣa's Sacrifice," particularly those that emphasize the death of Satī and the subsequent establishment of the *śāktapīṭhas*—see D. C. Sircar, *The Śākta Pīṭhas*, 2nd ed. (Delhi: Motilal Banarsidass, 1973), 6; O'Flaherty, *Hindu Myths*, 251; Cornelia Dimmit and J. A. B. van Buitenen, *Classical Hindu Mythology: A Reader in the Sanskrit Purāṇas* (Philadelphia: Temple University Press, 1978), 174–179. That said, neither Cakrapāṇidatta nor the classical medical *saṃhitā*s refer to the child of Rudra's anger as Vīrabhadra.

19. Ci 3.14–25.

20. Commentary on CS Ci 3.27: imminent causes (*pratyāsanna*) are described at CS Ni 1.17, and more distant causes (*vyavahita*) are described at CS Ni 1.19, 25, 29.

21. CS Ci 3.12: "Fever does not seize an embodied creature that is *nirdoṣaṃ*"—*nirdoṣaṃ* means "without doṣa (humor)" as well as "faultless." This dual meaning is well-suited to the melding of biophysical (humoral) and socioethical (ritually culpable) causes and effects in the narrative accounts of *jvara*.

22. On the modern-day perceived socioreligious causes and effects of leprosy, vitiligo, and associated skin diseases in the city of Banaras, and India in general, see Ronald L. Barrett, *Aghor Medicine: Pollution, Death, and Healing in Northern India* (Berkeley: University of California Press, 2008).

23. Wendy Doniger, "Minimyths and Maximyths and Political Points of View," in *Myth and Method*, ed. Laurie L. Patton and Wendy Doniger (Charlottesville: University Press of Virginia, 1996).

24. Doniger, "Minimyths and Maximyths," 116–118.
25. CS Ni 1.35.
26. BS Ci 2.1–3, 8.
27. SS Ut 39.9–13.
28. AHS Ni 2.1–2.
29. MN Jvaranidāna 2.1.
30. Outside of Indian textual studies, perhaps the most widely known practice of textual chronological estimation with the basic rule of thumb that the shortest of similar narratives was composed first is found among scholars of the three synoptic Gospels of the New Testament. The Gospel of Mark, the shortest of the three texts, is generally considered by Biblical scholars to have been composed first (ca. 95 C.E.), and its basic, bare-bones story lines were later adopted and expanded in the Gospels of Matthew and Luke.
31. See also BS Ci 1.1–2, where the *Bhelasaṃhitā* briefly recaps the *Carakasaṃhitā*'s account of fever and "Dakṣa's Sacrifice."
32. AV 5.30.8, 9; 9.8.5.
33. Filliozat, *The Classical Doctrine*, 121, fn. 2.
34. The presence of assonance between *takmán* and *ātaṅka* is justly open to discussion (cf. the indisputable assonance in the English words "feign," "gain," and "same," for instance, which have identical vowel sounds but differing surrounding consonant sounds).
35. YS 3.245; *Śakuntalā* 3.66 (Monier-Williams edition) and *Abhijñāna-śākuntalam* 3.12 (Karmarkar edition).
36. CS Ci 3.296–316.
37. Zysk, *Medicine in the Veda*, 34.
38. Zysk, "Fever in Vedic India," 617; Zysk, *Medicine in the Veda*, 34, 41–42; Filliozat, *The Classical Doctrine*, 116–117.
39. Regarding Hrūḍu—AV 1.25.2–3; Agni—AV 1.25.1, 6.20.1–2; Varuṇa—AV 1.25.3; Rudra—AV 11.2.22, 26.
40. AV 5.22.6; 11.2.22, 26.
41. AV 5.22.12: takmanbhrātrā balāsena svasrā kāsikayā saha / pāmnā bhrātṛvyeṇa saha gachāmum araṇaṃ janam.
42. Sharma, *Āyurved kā Vaijñānik Itihās*, 27.
43. AV 1.25.1–4; 6.20.1–3. In the first of these two invocations to Takman, we encounter the epithet Hrūḍu. Kenneth Zysk has suggested this esoteric name is the "secret key" a knowledgeable physician would use to appease Takman and ultimately encourage him to leave the patient (*Medicine in the Veda*, 37).
44. AV 5.22.5, 8–9. In these three verses, Takman's home (*okas*) is said to be among the Mūjavant people (who live in the Mūjavat mountains) and among the Mahāvṛṣa ("Great Bull") people; he "belongs to" or is "fit for" (*nyocara*) the region of the Bālhīkas. Moreover, Takman and the peoples of these regions are "connected" as kin (*bandhu*).
45. AV 1.22.4; 7.116.2.
46. Zysk, *Medicine in the Veda*, 9.
47. On the *Bhelasaṃhitā* and its relationship to the compendium of Caraka and the Vedas, see Sharma, *Āyurved kā Vaijñānik Itihās*, 237–239;

P. V. Sharma, "Other Compendia of *Bhela, Kāśyapa,* and *Hārīta,*" in *History of Indian Medicine,* 223–225; Tsutomu Yamashita, "Towards a Critical Edition of the *Bhelasaṃhitā,*" *Journal of the European Ayurvedic Society,* 5 (1997): 19–24.

48. Wendy Doniger O'Flaherty, *The Origins of Evil in Hindu Mythology* (Berkeley: University of California Press, 1976, 6.

49. O'Flaherty, *The Origins of Evil,* 7.

50. Similarly, Rahul Peter Das has noted the moral component of leprosy (*kuṣṭha*) in the *Suśrutasaṃhitā* ("Notions of 'Contagion' in Classical Indian Medical Texts," in *Contagion: Perspectives from Pre-Modern Societies,* ed. Lawrence I. Conrad and Dominik Wujastyk [Aldershot: Ashgate Publishing, 2000], 73).

51. The Four Cosmic ages (*yugas*) are: [1] Satya or Kṛta, [2] Tretā, [3] Dvāpara, and [4] Kali.

52. On the social conditions of the different *yugas* in nonmedical literature, see especially MP 165; on the state of the Satya (Kṛta) Yuga, see VāP 8.32–67, 99.413 and BrṇḍP 2.7.21, 45–49; on the state of dharma in the Tretā Yuga, see VāP 57.81–125.

53. CS Vi 3.24–27.

54. CS Vi 3.24.

55. Commentary on CS Ci 3.14–25.

56. Romila Thapar, *Time as a Metaphor of History: The Krishna Bharadwaj Memorial Lecture* (New Delhi: Oxford University Press, 1996), 25.

57. Thapar, *Time as Metaphor,* 13–19.

58. Palmyr Cordier, *Étude sur la Médecine Hindoue: (Temps Védiques et Héroiques),* Thèse pour le Doctorat en Médecine, Faculté de Médecine et de Pharmacie de Bordeaux (Paris: A. Bellier et Ce., 1894), 30–31.

59. On Śiva and the sublimation and release of sexual activity, see Sudhir Kakar, *The Inner World: A Psycho-analytic Study of Childhood and Society in India,* 2nd ed. (Delhi: Oxford University Press, 1981), 23–24. A particularly vivid portrait of Śiva the "great yogi" (*mahāyogin*), whose powers for maintaining celibacy are unexcelled, may be read at BhP 1.12.23; 15.12; 18.14.

60. Kenneth G. Zysk, "Does Ancient Indian Medicine Have a Theory of Contagion?," in *Contagion,* 88–89.

61. ṚV 10.61-5–9.

62. Here I summarize the stories found in ŚB, Mādhyandina 1.7.4.1–8, Kāṇva 2.7.2.1–8, 1.1.2.5–6 and AB 3.33–34.

63. Maurice Bloomfield, *The Atharva-Veda and the Gopatha-Brāhmaṇa: Grundriss der Indo-Arischen Philologie und Altertumskunde* (Strassburg: Verlag von Karl J. Trübner, 1899), 118.

64. MBh 12.283.16–33. See also Sircar, *The Śākta Pīṭhas,* 5–6.

65. BhP 4.2–7; BrāP 39; KP 1.15.1–81; *Kumārasambhava* 1.21; PP 1.5.1–96; ŚP 2.16–43.

66. For example, Dakṣa disparages Rudra-Śiva for being a naked mendicant who carries a human skull for a begging bowl; he also points out to the sage Dadhīca that his son-in-law is Rudra, the destroyer, not Śiva, the auspicious one, and therefore not deserving of a portion of the sacrifice.

67. This myth has been recognized as an early depiction of so-called widow-burning, *satī*.

68. E.g., BhP 4.5; 7.17; VāP 30.130–160, 101.299; KP 1.14.4–97.

69. Sircar, *The Śākta Pīṭhas*, 6–7.

70. Mitchell Weiss, "Caraka Saṃhitā on the Doctrine of Karma," in *Karma and Rebirth*, 110–115.

71. Weiss, "Caraka Saṃhitā on the Doctrine of Karma," 110.

72. CS Ci 3.26. Incidentally, in personal conversations with colleagues at the World Sanskrit Conference in Kyoto, Japan, in 2009, I learned that the presence of fever at the moment of birth is a common theme in many cultures throughout the world; fever at death is not as common, however.

73. Although the embryological passages in the *Mārkaṇḍeya Purāṇa* postdate the *Carakasaṃhitā*, *Mārkaṇḍeya*'s use of the concept *tamas* in reference to experiences at the beginning of life are strikingly similar to *Caraka*'s use of the term. These passages are therefore helpful in the analysis of the medical literature. Although it is possible that the compilers of the *Mārkaṇḍeya Purāṇa* borrowed and elaborated the association of *tamas* with birth from the *Carakasaṃhitā*, this is not a question that I can pursue here.

74. MāP 10.1–7, 48–95; 11.1–32.

75. For instance, see MāP 11.19. The *Garbha Upaniṣad* is a seminal text for both later ayurvedic and non-ayurvedic speculations on the formation and development of the human body. See Lakshmi Kapani's useful, if brief, introduction to and translation of the *Garbha Upaniṣad*: "Note on the Garbha-Upaniṣad" and "Upaniṣad of the Embryo." Rahul Peter Das's *The Origin of the Life of a Human Being: Conception and the Female According to Ancient Indian Medical and Sexological Literature* (Delhi: Motilal Banarsidass, 2003) is perhaps the most exhaustive and wide-ranging, in terms of the literature discussed, source for the textual history, both medical and nonmedical, on the origins of human life.

76. CS Śā 6.24.

77. Minoru Hara, "A Note on the Buddha's Birth Story," in *Indianisme et Bouddhisme: Mélanges offerts à Mgr Étienne Lamotte* (Louvain: Université Catholique de Louvain, 1980), 149.

Notes to Chapter 4

1. Marcel Mauss, "Techniques of the Body," trans. Ben Brewster, *Economy and Society*, vol. 2, no. 1 (February 1973): 85.

2. I also address the context of the *Kāśyapasaṃhitā* in "Calculating Fecundity in the *Kāśyapa Saṃhitā*," in *Health and Religious Rituals in South Asia: Disease, Possession, and Healing*, ed. Fabrizio Ferrari (London: Routledge, 2011), 114–126.

3. Muelenbeld, *HIML*, IIA: 25.

4. Wujastyk has noted that the *Bhelasaṃhitā* covers a lot of the same material as, and likely dates from a period close in time to, the *Carakasaṃhitā*;

it survives today, he says, "in a single problematic manuscript" (*Roots of Ayurveda*, xxx, fn. 16). For more on the contents and history of the *Bhelasaṃhitā*, see Yamashita, "Towards a Critical Edition of the Bhelasaṃhitā"; Sharma, "Other Compendia of *Bhela, Kāśyapa*, and *Hārīta*," 223–225; and K. H. Krishnamurthy's introduction to *Bhela-Saṃhitā*, Sanskrit text with English translation, commentary and critical notes by K. H. Krishnamurthy, ed. P. V. Sharma, Haridāsa āyurveda sīrīja, 8 (Varanasi: Chaukhambha Visvabharati, 2000).

5. Meulenbeld, *HIML*, IIA: 27.

6. Meulenbeld, *HIML*, IIA: 39–41.

7. Wujastyk, *Roots of Ayurveda*, 164; see also Varier, *History of Ayurveda*, 131.

8. Wujastyk, *Roots of Ayurveda*, 163.

9. Sharma, *Āyurved kā Vaijñānik Itihās*, 153–154; Premvati V. Tewari, *Introduction to Kāśyapa-Saṃhitā* (Varanasi: Chaukhambha Visvabharati, 1997), 6. In this chapter I use the second of the two editions of the *Kāśyapasaṃhitā*, the 1938 Nepali edition, as well as Tewari's edition (*Kāśyapa-Saṃhitā or Vṛddhajīvakīya Tantra*, text with English translation and commentary by P. V. Tewari [Varanasi: Chaukhambha Visvabharati, 1996]).

10. Wujastyk translates the proper name, Vṛddhajīvaka, as "Old Lifegiver" (*Roots of Ayurveda*, 165, 179–182).

11. Sharma, *Āyurved kā Vaijñānik Itihās*, 164–169; Meulenbeld, *HIML*, IIA: 26; Tewari, introduction to *Kāśyapa-Saṃhitā or Vṛddhajīvakīya Tantra*, xiii–xiv; Girindranath Mukhopadhyaya, *History of Indian Medicine*, 3 vols., 1923 (reprint, New Delhi: Munshiram Manoharlal, 1994), III: 681–744; Zysk, *Asceticism and Healing*, 52–60.

12. Meulenbeld, *HIML*, IIA: 25; Sharma, *Āyurved kā Vaijñānik Itihās*, 153; Varier, *History of Ayurveda*, 119.

13. KS Kp 9.18–29.

14. Meulenbeld, *HIML*, IIA: 34.

15 See, for example, Wujastyk, *Roots of Ayurveda*, 163–189.

16. KS Kp 1.49–56.

17. KS Kp 2.7–12.

18. KS Kp 7.41–55.

19. AHS Śā 2.9–13; SS Ni 8.10; BS Śā 8.5; BVP Ci 70.72 (*garbhapāta*); SS Ni 8.9 and BS Sū 11.15 (*garbhacyuti*).

20. Ḍalhaṇa's commentary on SS Śā 10.57.

21. AHS Śā 2.15–18ab; SS Śā 10.57 (*nāgodara garbha*); AHS Śā 18cd–21ab (*līnagarbha*).

22. AHS Śā 2, Ut 33.28–52.

23. KS Sū 22.14. In her translation of the *Kāśyapasaṃhitā*, Premvati Tewari translates *garbhacyavana* as "abortion." This translation would indicate that either the shaking of the embryo is deliberative and/or the falling of the embryo is the intended outcome of an act done to the pregnant woman.

24. KS Kh 10.161 and KS Si 1.41.

25. KS Kh 10.168–169, 175.

26. Premvati Tewari, *Āyurvedīya Prasūtitantra Evaṃ Strītoga*, 2 vols., 3rd ed. (Varanasi: Chaukhambha Orientalia, 2003), I: 476.

27. Wujastyk emends the text here from the gerund *uṣitvā* to *aśitvā*, "having eaten" (from √aś—*Roots of Ayurveda*, 169). He uses the Śarmā 1988 edition (*Roots of Ayurveda*, 164); I use the Śarmā 1938 edition. On my reading, there is no need to alter the text. It is entirely in keeping with ayurvedic parlance to use the term *uṣitvā*, "having burned" (from √uṣ), to indicate the process of digestion (known as *vipāka*, literally "ripe; ripening, cooking"), which is conceived of as a process of cooking (*pācana, dīpana*) food in the body's digestive fire (*pācakāgni* and *jaṭharāgni*).

28. This is a reference to the myth of the churning of the Ocean of Milk, out of which the nectar of immortality (*amṛta*) emerged, along with many other things, such as the divine physician Dhanvantari and the system of Āyurveda itself (MBh 1.15.5–13, 1.16.1–40, 1.17.1–30; VP 1.9.2–116; see also O'Flaherty, *Hindu Myths*, 273–279; Dimmitt and van Buitenen, *Classical Hindu Mythology*, 94–98).

29. Wujastyk (*Roots of Ayurveda*, 170, fn. 9) gives a brief synopsis of Dīrghajihvī as well as secondary literature on her activities in Vedic literature; O'Flaherty (*Tales of Sex and Violence: Folklore, Sacrifice, and Danger in the Jaiminīya Brāhmaṇa* [Chicago: University of Chicago Press, 1985], 101–103) discusses Dīrghajihvī in the *Jaiminīya Brāhmaṇa*, in which she is depicted in a much more highly sexualized aspect than we find her in the *Kāśyapasaṃhitā*.

30. These are three groups of deities—eight Vasus, eleven Rudras, twelve Ādityas—from Vedic mythology that, along with the two Aśvins, make up the so-called "thirty-three gods" (O'Flaherty, *Hindu Myths*, 39, fn. 25; Wujastyk, *Roots of Ayurveda*, 170, fn. 10).

31. KS Kp 6. 1–6.

32. KS Kp 6.

33. KS Kp 7.

34. BhP 9.3; Revatī also appears as the wife of Balarāma in the *Harivaṃśa, Śiśupālavadham*, and *Meghadūta*.

35. TS 4.4.10.3; MS 2.13.20, 166.8; KauS 39.13.

36. BṛhS 15.25.

37. Patrick Olivelle, trans., *Upaniṣads* (New York: Oxford University Press, 1996), 114.

38. MBh Vanaparvan 219.28; AHS Ut 3.27b–32a; SS Ut 27.3.

39. See Jean Filliozat, *Etude de démonologie indienne. Le Kumāratantra de Rāvaṇa et les textes parallèles indiens, tibétains, chinois, cambodgien et arabe* (Paris: Imprimerie Nationale, 1937), 19–20; Bhagwan Dash and Lalitesh Kasyap, *Five Specialised Therapies of Ayurveda (Pañca-karma)* (New Delhi: Concept Publishing Company, 1992), 114–126; Wujastyk, *Roots of Ayurveda*, 175–177.

40. David Gordon White, *Kiss of the Yoginī: "Tantric Sex" in Its South Asian Contexts* (Chicago: University of Chicago Press, 2003), 34–36.

41. MāP 51.105–107.

42. Dominik Wujastyk, "Miscarriages of Justice: Demonic Vengeance in Classical Indian Medicine," in *Religion, Health, and Suffering*, ed. J. Hinnels and R. Porter (London: Kegan Paul International, 1999), 267–270 and *Roots of Ayurveda*, 165–185.

43. See Premvati Tewari's three works: *Kāśyapa-Saṃhitā or Vṛddhajīvakīya Tantra; Introduction to Kāśyapa-Saṃhitā;* and *Āyurvedīya Prasūtitantra Evaṃ Strītoga.*

44. Geri Malandra, *Unfolding a Maṇḍala: The Buddhist Cave Temples at Ellora* (Albany: State University of New York Press, 1993), 104–105.

45. Zysk, *Asceticism and Healing*, 26–29.

46. Malandra, *Unfolding a Maṇḍala*, 103.

47. Malandra, *Unfolding a Maṇḍala*, 104.

48. White, *Kiss of the Yoginī*, 64.

49. KS Kp 6.62–69.

50. KS Kp 6.30cd–31ab

51. Tewari, introduction to *Kāśyapa-Saṃhitā or Vṛddhajīvakīya Tantra*, xxix.

52. See Cerulli, "Calculating Fecundity," 116–119.

53. Pilipicchikā is the name of one of the mothers (*mātṛkās*) associated with child possession and seizures, also known as the Twleve Skanda-Seizers: Nandanā, Sunandā, Putanā, Mukhamaṇḍikā, Kaṭapūtanā, Śakunikā, Śuṣkarevatī, Aryakā, Bhūsūtikā, Nirṛtā, Pilipicchikā, and Kāmukā. See Filliozat, *Etude de démonologie indienne*, 19–20.

54. KS Kp 6.7.

55. KS Kp 6.8.

56. Cerulli, "Religio-Medical Perspectives on the Body," forthcoming.

57. KS Kp 6.65–66.

58. E.g., CS Vi 8.94.

59. See especially Roland Barthes, *Mythologies*, trans. Annette Lavers (New York: Hill and Wang, 1972) and Claude Lévi-Strauss, *The Jealous Potter* (Chicago: University of Chicago Press, 1988).

60. See, for example, Manu 9.26.

61. On this issue, not all Brāhmaṇas agree. Charles Malamoud has pointed out that the *Taittirīya Brāhmaṇa* says only brahmin men are born with these three debts. The *Śatapatha Brāhmaṇa*, however, claims that every man is born with these three debts, plus a fourth, to his fellow men. The *Śatapatha Brāhmaṇa* consequently presents a problem for many men: if all men are born debtors, only some of them are capable of settling their life accounts, for only twice-born men can study the Vedas (via the *upanayana* rite); and only those men who have studied the Vedas and received the *upanayana* thread are allowed to perform the sacrifice (Charles Malamoud, *Cooking the World: Ritual & Thought in Ancient India*, trans. David White (Delhi: Oxford University Press, 1996), 96–97.

62. MBh 1.111.10–17.

63. The meaning of immortality with regard to the *śrāddha* rites seems to have included two different connotations from the time of the Vedas, a tension "built in from the very beginning, a simple tension between the desire to

prevent rebirth and the desire to assure rebirth" (Wendy Doniger O'Flaherty, "Karma and Rebirth in the Vedas and Purāṇas," in *Karma and Rebirth*, 4). The prevention of rebirth meant that one's father would not suffer "repeated death" (*punarmṛtyu*) from life to life in *saṃsāra*. This concern is elaborated in the Upaniṣads. In view of the idea that renewable existence only leads to repeated death, the Upaniṣads develop the notion that the only ultimately worthwhile goal must involve a complete break in the cycle of birth and death, hence *mokṣa*, "release" from the cycle of rebirth and redeath.

64. KS Kp 6.12b–13a.

65. Zysk, "Does Ancient Indian Medicine Have a Theory of Contagion," in *Contagion* 88; Das, "Notions of Contagion," in *Contagion* 65–66, 72.

66. Wendy Doniger and Sudhir Kakar, introduction to their translation, *Kamasutra* (Oxford: Oxford University Press, 2002), xxxi.

67. Brian Smith, *Classifying the Universe: The Ancient Indian Varṇa System and the Origins of Caste* (Oxford: Oxford University Press, 1994) 86–88.

68. A. Stewart Woodburne, "The Evil Eye in South Indian Folklore," in *The Evil Eye: A*

Casebook, ed. Alan Dundes (Madison: University of Wisconsin Press, 1981), 56–57.

69. KS Kp 6.8.

70. KS Kp 6.25–30.

71. Zysk, *Asceticism and Healing*, 15.

72. It is worth pointing out here, as I will again at length in Chapter 7, my hermeneutical tack in this book deliberately sidesteps the long-held arguments in the history of Indian medicine, seen in works over the past three decades, that morally didactic material in ayurvedic literature was cleverly incorporated into ostensibly "scientific" compendia with the purpose of establishing these sources squarely in the brahminic traditions. One can find examples of this line of argument in Basham, "The Practice of Medicine" and Chattopadhyaya, "Tradition of Rationalist Medicine." Contrastingly, Steven Engler has offered ("'Science' vs. 'Religion") a useful analysis of the anachronistic reading of the modern science-religion debate into the Sanskrit medical classics among historians of Indian medicine (and in the history of medicine in general); he productively attempts to situate, as I do here, Āyurveda within the human sciences, broadly conceived, as a important Indian knowledge system that was equally impacted by historical social forces, such as religion and economics, and a contributor to those forces.

73. Martha Ann Selby, "Narratives of Conception, Gestation, and Labour in Sanskrit Ayurvedic Texts," *Asian Medicine: Tradition and Modernity*, vol. 1, no. 2 (2005): 270–271.

74. Selby, "Narratives of Conception," 272.

75. Selby, "Narratives of Conception," 273.

76. Selby, "Narratives of Conception," 273.

77. CS Śā 4.14.

78. CS and AHS designate the third month, whereas SS and BVP mark the fourth month, as the onset of double-heartedness (Tewari, *Āyurvedīya Prasūtitantra Evaṃ Strītoga*, I: 206–207).

79. CS Śā 4.15–19; SS Śā 3.18; AHS Śā 1; ASS Śā 2.19–21.
80. CS Śā 4.17.
81. KS Śā 5.12–15.

Notes to Chapter 5

1. ṚV 10.161.1; AV 3.11.1. For stand-alone references to *yakṣma*, see ṚV 10.85.31 and AV 9.8.10.

2. Filliozat, *The Classical Doctrine*, 99–100; Zysk, *Medicine in the Veda*, 12–17.

3. *Amarakośa* 2.6.51.

4. For instance, Monier-Williams, *Sanskrit-English Dictionary*, and Apte, *Practical Sanskrit-English Dictionary*, s.v. "rājayakṣman."

5. Mario Vallauri, introduction to *Jīvānandana (La Felicità Dell' Anima) di Ānandarāyamakhin* (Lanciano: G. Carabba, 1929), iv.

6. Filliozat, *The Classical Doctrine*, 100.

7. SS Ut 41.1–5; BS 4; AHS Ni 5.1–4; ASS Ci 7.1, Ut 50.178; CS Ni 6.12, 8.11–14.

8. CS Ci 8.1–13.

9. The word "scrofula" literally means "little sow" (a diminutive of the Latin *scrōfa*, "breeding sow").

10. René and Jean Dubos, *The White Plague: Tuberculosis, Man, and Society*, 1952 (reprint, New Brunswick: Rutgers University Press, 1987), 7–8.

11. Thomas Dormandy, *The White Death: A History of Tuberculosis* (New York: New York University Press, 2000), 4–5; Frank Ryan, *The Forgotten Plague: How the Battle against Tuberculosis Was Won—and Lost* (Boston: Little, Brown and Company, 1992), 6–7.

12. ṚV 10.85.2: somen' ādityā balinaḥ / somena pṛthivī mahī / atho nakṣatrāṇām eṣām / upasthe soma ahitaḥ.

13. V. S. Apte, *Practical Sanskrit-English Dictionary*. 4th ed. (Delhi: Motilal Banarsidass, 2004) and Monier-Williams, *Sanskrit-English Dictionary*, s.v. "upastha." See also Filliozat, *The Classical Doctrine*, 101.

14. AV 19.7.2; MS 2.2.7; KṭhS 11.3. The daughter of the Sun, Sūryā, in the *Atharvaveda* is the constellation Rohiṇī. About this shift from Sūryā to Rohiṇī, Filliozat wrote: "An assimilation has, therefore, taken place between Sūryā and Rohiṇī, the two feminine Suns" (*The Classical Doctrine*, 101).

15. TS 2.3.5.1–3.

16. Zysk, *Medicine in the Veda*, 12.

17. KālP 20.104–106, 21.49–50.

18. David Gordon White, *The Alchemical Body*, 24.

19. Zysk, *Medicine in the Veda*, 15.

20. White, *The Alchemical Body*, 25.

21. Louise Lacey, *Lunaception: A Feminine Odyssey into Fertility and Contraception* (New York: Coward, McCann, and Geoghegen, 1975).

22. Wendy Doniger O'Flaherty, *Women, Androgynes, and Other Mythical Beasts* (Chicago: University of Chicago Press, 1980), 44 and *Śiva: The Erotic Ascetic*, 55, 261–262.

23. For an explanation of the sources of male and female "śukra," see Ḍalhaṇa's commentary on SS Sū 14.10.

24. SS Sū 14.10.

25. To date, the best study of *kalā* in Sanskrit literature is Jan Gonda's "The Number Sixteen," in *Change and Continuity in Indian Religion*, 1965 (reprint, New Delhi: Munshiram Manoharlal, 1997), 115–130. On the duration of the *kalā* and lunar month in the medical context, see Wujastyk *Roots of Ayurveda*, 111, fn. 61.

26. SS Sū 14.14–15.

27. Commentary on CS Ci 8.38–47.

28. On potency therapy in classical Indian medicine, see Kenneth G. Zysk, "Potency Therapy in Classical Indian Medicine," *Asian Medicine: Tradition and Modernity*, vol. 1, no. 1 (2005): 101–118.

29. Commentary on CS Ci 8.1–13.

30. G. Jan Meulenbeld, "The Woes of *Ojas* in the Modern World," in *Modern and Global Ayurveda: Pluralism and Paradigms*, ed. Dagmar Wujastyk and Frederick M. Smith (Albany: State University of New York, 2008), 160.

31. Meulenbeld, "The Woes of *Ojas*," 168–169.

32. Commentary on CS Sū 28.4; cf. SS Sū 15.19.

33. Gonda, *Change and Continuity*, 42.

34. Zimmermann, "Ṛtu-Sātmya," 102.

35. CS Ni 6.12.

36. Sheldon Pollock, "Rāmāyaṇa and Political Imagination in India," *Journal of Asian Studies*, vol. 52, no. 2 (May 1993): 282.

37. RĀM 4.18.37–38, cited in Pollock, "Rāmāyaṇa and Political Imagination," 282.

38. MBh Āraṇyaka Parvan 24.10; 26.14, 15; 80.106; 132.1; 173.3; 180.32; 190.73; 253.10; Virāṭa Parvan 7.7; 24.13; 63.15; Udyoga Parvan 27.14; Bhīṣma Parvan 20.3, 20; Droṇa Parvan 138.34; Karṇa Parvan 4.97, 104; 5.1; 54.5; Śalya Parvan 61.33; Śānti Parvan 280.23; Anuśāsana Parvan 96.6; 105.25; Aśvamedha Parvan 10.16, 23, 27, 35; Mahāprasthānika Parvan 3.16.

39. MBh Śānti Parvan 68.39–47; 92.1, 38–41.

40. J. C. Heesterman, *The Ancient Indian Royal Consecration: The Rājasūya Described according to the Yajus Texts*, Disputationes Rheno-trajectinae 2 ('s-Gravenhage: Mouton, 1957), 10, 223–224. On the royal duty of kings, see Patrick Olivelle, *The Āśrama System: The History and Hermeneutics of a Religious Institution*, 1993 (reprint, New Delhi: Munshiram Manoharlal, 2004), 201–204.

41. Sharma has described the view of kṣatriya dharma in the *Suśrutasaṃhitā* within a larger discussion of *Suśruta*'s statements on class (*varṇa*), caste (*jāti*), and stage of life (*āśrama—Āyurved kā Vaijñānik Itihās*, 70–74).

42. Zimmermann, *The Jungle and the Aroma of Meats*, 181 (emphasis in original).

43. SS Sū 34: yuktasenīyam adhyāyaṃ.

44. On governance: Manu 7.2–3, 35, 110–112; 8.172, 303–309; 9.253. On battle: Manu 7.87–95, 184–200; 10.119. On a heroic death: Manu 9.323.

45. Manu 7.79, 145.

46. Stephanie Jamison, *Sacrificed Wife/Sacrificer's Wife: Women, Ritual, and Hospitality in Ancient India* (Oxford: Oxford University Press, 1996), 195–199.

47. Commentary on CS Ci 8.10.

48. CS Ci 8.24.

49. On the importance of self-knowledge, *ātmajñāna*, for bodily and mental health in the *Carakasaṃhitā* and Cakrapāṇidatta's *Āyurvedadīpikā*, see Cerulli and Brahmadathan, "Know Thy Body," 103–105.

50. CS Sū 25.40.

51. CS Śā 5.8.

52. Wujastyk ("Medicine and Dharma," 834) and Zimmermann (*The Jungle and the Aroma of Meats*, 190) have looked at the concepts of *pravṛtti* and *nivṛtti* in Āyurveda as they pertain specifically to vegetarianism and *ahiṃsā* ("non-injury").

Notes to Chapter 6

1. Dominik Wujastyk has suggested that Venkojī might have died as late as 1687 ("The Questions of King Tukkoji: Medicine at an Eighteenth Century South Indian Court," *Indian Journal of History of Science* 41.4 [2006], 362). Heinrich Zimmer mistakenly dated of the *Jīvānandanam* (which he translated as "The Bliss of the Life-Monad or Soul") to the first half of the seventeenth century (*Hindu Medicine*, 61).

2. The same ambiguity over authorship looms over another allegorical drama regularly attributed to Ānandarāya, *The Nuptials of Knowledge* (*Vidyāpariṇayam*).

3. T. S. Kuppuswami Sastri, "Ramabhadra-Dikshita and the Southern Poets of His Time," *Indian Antiquary*, vol. 33 (May 1904): 181; K. R. Subramanian, *The Maratha Rajas of Tanjore* (Madras: K. R. Subramanian, 1928), 32–33; V. Raghavan, *Śāhendravilāsa (A Poem on the Life of King Śāhaji of Tanjore, 1684–1710) of Śrīdhara Veṅkaṭeśa (Ayyāvāl)*, Tanjore Saraswati Mahal Series no. 54 (Tiruchi: The Kalyan Press, 1952), 29; I. Shekhar, *Sanskrit Drama: Its Origin and Decline* (Leiden: E.J. Brill, 1960), 172, fn. 7; Meulenbeld, *HIML*, IIA: 345.

4. Unless otherwise noted, I use Aiyangar's edition, *Jīvānandanam: Āyurvedaśātattvaprakaṭanaparaṃ prācīnaṃ nāṭakam*, ed. with a Sanskrit commentary by M. Duraiswami Aiyangar (Madras: Adyar Library, 1947).

5. This is research into which I am currently looking in coordination with a full English translation of the *Jīvānandanam*. To date, there have been only two translations of the *Jīvānandanam* into European languages, one in Italian (Vallauri, *Jīvānandana [La Felicità Dell' Anima]*, 1929) and one in German (Adolf Weckerling, *Das Glück des Lebens: Medizinisches Drama von Ânandarâyamakhî* [Greifswald: Universitätsverlag Ratsbuchhandlung L. Bamberg, 1937]).

6. Zimmer, *Hindu Medicine*, 61–62.

7. Weckerling, introduction to *Das Glück des Lebens*, 36–38; Maria Schetelich, "Niti in Anandarayamakhis Drama 'Jivanandana,'" *Altorientalische Forschungen* 11.2 (1984): 300–302.

8. Vallauri, introduction to *Jīvānandana (La Felicità Dell' Anima)*, vii–xiv.

9. Sheldon Pollock and the contributors to the "Sanskrit Knowledge Systems on the Eve of Colonialism Project" (2001–04) have skillfully documented the richness and diversity of Sanskrit literature during this period—http://www.columbia.edu/itc/mealac/pollock/sks/index.html

10. Saroja Agravāla, *Prabodhacandrodaya aur uskī Hindī paramparā*. Āgarā Viśvavidyālaya kī Ph.D. (Prayāj: Hindī Sāhitya Sammelan, 1962).

11. Kapstein (trans., *The Rise of Wisdom Moon by Krishna-mishra* [New York: New York University Press and JJC Foundation, 2009], xxxii–xxxiii, lviii fn. 7) cites the following work as an example of a literary critic using the term *pratīkanāṭaka* in the sense of allegory: Gāyatrī Devī Bakhśī, *Saṃskṛt ke pratīk nāṭak ke rūp meṃ śrī Vedāntadeśika kṛt Saṃkalpasūryodaya ek adhyayan* (Jaipur: Saṃghī Prakāśan, 1993).

12. Compare *samāsokti* with *upalakṣaṇa*: "the act of implying something that has not been expressed, implying any analogous object where only one is specified; using a term metaphorically or elliptically or in a generic sense; synecdoche (of a part for the whole, of an individual for the species, or of a quality for that in which it resides)" (Monier-Williams, *Sanskrit-English Dictionary*, s.v. "upalakṣaṇa").

13. Pollock, *The Language of the Gods*, 361.

14. Kapstein, *The Rise of Wisdom Moon*, xxxiv.

15. Ānandarāya's play at times reads like a sustained, seven-act "simultaneous narration" (*śleṣa*), which, according to Yigal Bronner, "typically involves a metamorphosis of the entire utterance—nouns, verbs, and prepositions—in a way that creates a new sentence with a new vocabulary, a new syntax, and, obviously, a new meaning" (*Extreme Poetry: The South Asian Movement of Simultaneous Narration* [New York: Columbia University Press, 2010], 181).

16. I have also summarized Ānandarāya's play in "The Joy of Life: Medicine, Politics, and Religion," in *Medical Texts and Manuscripts in Indian Cultural History*, ed. Anthony Cerulli, Karin Preisendanz, and Dominik Wujastyk (New Delhi: Manohar Publishers, forthcoming).

17. JVM 1.6–8.

18. Clifford Geertz, *The Interpretation of Cultures* (New York: Basic Books, 1973), 93–94.

19. Lupton, *Medicine as Culture*, 69.

20. BG 2.31–33.

21. Schetelich, "Niti in Anandarayamakhis Drama," 300, fn. 7.

22. JVM 3.8–9.

23. JVM 4.24.

24. Greg Bailey, *Materials for the Study of Ancient Indian Ideologies:* pravṛtti *and* nivṛtti (Torino: Indologica Taurinensia, 1985), 17–22.

25. Greg Bailey, "The *pravṛtti/nivṛtti* project at La Trobe University with Notes on the Meaning of *vṛt* in the *Bhagavadgītā*," *Indologica Taurinensia*,

29 (2003): 13. Citing Bailey's 1985 *pravṛtti-nivṛtti* study, Matthew Kapstein recently criticized the characterization of *pravṛtti* and *nivṛtti* as independent ideologies, arguing instead that they are "complementary facets of a common ideology" (introduction to *The Rise of Wisdom Moon*, lix, fn. 13).

26. For this term, *vasā*, in his commentary Aiyangar cites the SS (without providing a specific reference): śuddhamāṃsasya yaḥ snehaḥ sā vasāparikīrtitā.

27. This octet is unusual, fitting as it does somewhere between the typical seven or ten bodily constituents (*dhātus*): chyle, blood, flesh, fat, bone, marrow, semen (plus three: hair, skin, sinews).

28. JVM 6.12–13.

29. JVM 6.19.

30. JVM 6.29. Here the text reads *mokṣa* for "release" and *śilpaśāstra* for "matters of this world." For the latter translation, I follow Aiyangar's commentary, where he interprets Ānandarāya's use of *śilpaśāstra* to mean practical matters in general and the first three *puruṣārthas*—kāma, artha, and dharma—in particular.

31. JVM 7.28–29.

32. Cf. MBh Vanaparvan, 83.83; VāP, 77.55; BrṇḍP, 3.13.56. For variants of "puṇḍarīkapuram" (and similar compounds) in Sanskrit literature, also see *Śabdakalpadruma* 3.164–165.

33. MP 22.77.

34. VP 24.51.

35. Carl Cappeller, "Ein Medizinisches Sanskritdrama," in *Festschrift für Ernst Windisch* (Leipzig: Harrassowitz, 1914), 109.

Notes to Chapter 7

1. Wujastyk, "Medicine and Dharma," 838.

2. Commentary on CS Sū 1.43.

3. SS Sū 35.

4. Paul Veyne, *Did the Greeks Believe in Their Myths: An Essay on the Constitutive Imagination*, trans. Paula Wissing (Chicago: University of Chicago Press, 1988), 14.

5. Veyne, *Did the Greeks Believe in Their Myths*, 18.

6. To note just three examples: looking at the historical development of classical Indian medicine, Kenneth Zysk frequently used the phrase "magico-religious medicine" vis-à-vis "empirico-rational medicine" (*Asceticism and Healing*); Arion Roşu has done work on what he calls "magic squares" (*les carrés magiques*) in Āyurveda ("Etudes âyurvédiques III"); and Julius Jolly frequently refers to magic, sorcery, and folk medicine in his history of Āyurveda (*Indian Medicine*).

7. Engler, "'Science' vs. 'Religion,'" 417.

8. E.g., *pramehin*: CS Sū 1.13.91, 1.17.107; *atisārin*: SS Sū 1.29.69, 1.46.253; *gulmin*: AHS Ci 14.10, 78, 90.

9. CS Sū 9.3.

10. CS Sū 9.9.
11. Commentary on CS Sū 9.9.
12. CS Sū 11.54.
13. Basham, "The Practice of Medicine," 22.
14. Cerulli, "Religio-Medical Perspectives on the Body, Self, and Embodiment," forthcoming.
15. Sharma, *Āyurved kā Vaijñānik Itihās*, 517.
16. Sharma, *Āyurved kā Vaijñānik Itihās*, 517–523.
17. On the *pūrvapakṣin-uttarapakṣin* in the *bhāṣyas* of Patañjali and Vātsyāyana, see the reprints of Ramkrishna Gopal Bhandarkar's 1883 Wilson Lectures at the University of Bombay in Frits J. F. Staal, ed., *A Reader on the Sanskrit Grammarians* (Cambridge, MA: The MIT Press, 1972), 87–88, 94.

References

Primary Sources

Abhijñāna-Śākuntala of Kālidāsa. Edited by Raghunath Damodar Karmarkar. Reprint, Delhi: Chaukhamba Sanskrit Pratishthan, 2003.

Agnipurāṇa: A Collection of Hindu Mythology and Traditions. Edited by Rājendralāla Mitra. 3 vols. Bibliotheca Indica, no. 65. Reprint, Osnabrück: Biblio Verlag, 1985.

Aitareyabrāhmaṇam (Ṛgvedasya), with the commentary of Sāyaṇa Ācārya. Edited by Satyavrata Sāmaśramī. Calcutta: Satya Press, 1895.

Amarakośaḥ (Nāmaliṅgānuśāsanam) Śrīmadamarasiṃhaviracitaṃ. Edited with Hindi commentaries by Brahmananda Tripathi. Chaukhamba Surbharati-granthamala, no. 52. Benares: Chaukhamba Surbharati Prakashan, 1982.

Aṣṭāṅgahṛdayam, with the commentaries of Aruṇadatta and Hemādri. Edited by A. M. Kuṇṭe, K. R. S. Navare, and B. H. Parāḍakara. Jaikrishnadas Āyurveda series, no. 52. 9th ed. Varanasi: Chaukhambha Orientalia, 2002.

Aṣṭāṅgasaṃgraha, with Indu's Śaśilekhā commentary, notes, diagrams, appendices, and an English introduction by Bhagwan Dash. Edited by Rāmacandraśāstrī Kiñjavaḍekara. Delhi: Sri Satguru Publications, 1990.

Atharvavedasaṃhitā. Edited by R. Roth and W. D. Whitney. 3rd ed. Bonn: Ferd. Dümmlers Verlag, 1966.

Bhagavad Gita, with the commentary of Sri Sankaracharya. Edited and translated by Alladi Mahadeva Sastry. 13th ed. Madras: Samata Books, 2001.

Bhāgavatapurāṇa, with the commentary of Śrīdhara. Edited by J. L. Śāstrī. Delhi: Motilal Banarsidass, 1983.

Bhāvaprakāśḥ, nighaṇṭu yukta, Śrimadbhāvamiśrapraṇīta, savivaraṇa "Vidyotinī" Hindī vyākhyāpariśiṣṭasahitaḥ. Edited by Bhiṣagratna Śrī Brahmaśaṅkara Miśra. 2 vols. Kāśī Saṃskṛta-granthamālā, no. 130. 10th ed. Vārāṇasī: Caukhambhā Saṃskṛta Saṃsthāna, 2002.

Bhela-Saṃhitā. Sanskrit text with English translation, commentary and critical notes by K. H. Krishnamurthy. Edited by Priya Vrat Sharma. Haridāsa Āyurveda Sīrīja, no. 8. Varanasi: Chaukhambha Visvabharati, 2000.

Brahmāṇḍapurāṇa of Kṛṣṇa Dvaipāyana Vyāsa (containing introduction in Sanskrit and English and an alphabetical index of verses). Edited by J. L. Śāstrī. Delhi: Motilal Banrsidass, 1983.

Brahmamahāpurāṇam. Edited by Kṣmarāja Śrīkṛṣṇadāsa, Nāga-Śaraṇa Siṃha, and Rajendra-Nātha Śarmā. Delhi: Nag Publishers, 1985.

Bṛhatsaṃhitā Varāhamihiraviracitā. Paṇḍita Śrī Acyutānanda Jhā Śarmaṇā navīnodāharaṇopapattiyukta "Vimalā" Hindīṭīkayā sanāthīkṛtya saṃśodhana-purassaraṃ sampāditā. Vidyābhavana Saṃskṛta-granthamālā, no. 41. Reprint, Vārāṇasī: Caukhambā Vidyābhavana, 1997.

Carakasaṃhitā of Agniveśa, with the *Āyurvedadīpikā* of Cakrapāṇidatta. Edited by Jādavji Trikamji Āchārya. 5th ed. New Delhi: Munshiram Manoharlal, 1992.

Garuḍamahāpurāṇam. Edited by Nag Sharan Singh. Delhi: Nag Publishers, 1984.

Jīvānandanam Ānandarāyamakhipraṇītaṃ. Edited by Durgāprasāda Dvivedī and Kāśīnātha Pāṇḍuraṅga Paraba. Kāvyamāla, no. 27. Bombay: Nirṇaya Sāgara Press, 1891.

Jīvānandanam Śrīmadānandarāyamakhipraṇītaṃ, with an introduction by Paṇḍita Śrī Hariśāstrī Dādhīcaḥ. Edited by Paṇḍita Nārāyaṇadattavaidya. Khurja, U. P., 1933.

Jīvānandanam: Āyurvedaśātratattvaprakaṭanaparam prācīnaṃ nāṭakam. Ānandarāyamakhī praṇītam. Edited with a Sanskrit commentary by Duraiswami Aiyangar. Madras: Adyar Library, 1947.

Kālikāpurāṇe Mūrtivinirdeśaḥ. Edited by Biswanarayan Shastri. New Delhi: Indira Gandhi National Centre for the Arts, 1994.

Kāśyapasaṃhitā of Vṛddhajīvaka (microfiche). Edited by Vaidya Jādavjī Trikamjī Āchārya and Somanāth Śarma. Nepal Sanskrit series, no. 1. Kathmandu, 1938.

Kāśyapa-Saṃhitā or Vṛddhajīvakīya Tantra. Text with English translation and commentary by P. V. Tewari. Varanasi: Chaukhambha Visvabharati, 1996.

Kāṭhakam, die Saṃhitā der Kaṭha-çākhā. Edited by Leopold von Schroeder. 3 vols. Leipzig: F.A. Brockhaus, 1900–1910.

Kathāsaritsāgara of Somadevabhaṭṭa. Edited by Durgāprasāda Dvivedī and Kāśīnātha Pāṇḍuraṅga Paraba. Bombay: Nirṇaya Sāgara Press, 1889.

Kauçika-Sūtra of the Atharva Veda, with extracts from the commentaries of Dārila and Keçava. Edited by Maurice Bloomfield. New Haven: American Oriental Society, no. 14, 1890.

Kauṭilīya Arthśāstra. Edited by R. P. Kangle. 3 vols. 7th ed. Delhi: Motilal Banarsidass, 2000.

Kṛṣṇayajurvedīya-Taittirīya-saṃhitā. Sanskrit text with English translation by R. L. Kashyap. 3 vols. Bangalore: Sri Aurobindo Kapāli Sāstry Institute of Vedic Culture, 2002–2004.

Kumārasambhava. In *Works of Kālidāsa*, vol. 2, "Poetry." Sanskrit text with English translation by C. R. Devadhar. Delhi: Motilal Banarsidass, 1984.

Kūrmapurāṇa. Bombay: Lakṣmīveṅkaṭeśvara Press, 1926.

Mādhavanidānam (Rogaviniścaya) of Mādhavakara. Sanskrit text with English translation by K. R. Srikanta Murthy. Varanasi: Chaukhambha Orientalia, 1995.

Mahābhārata. Edited by V. S. Sukthankar, et al. 19 vols. Poona: Bhandarkar Oriental Research Institute, 1933–1959.

Maitrāyaṇī Saṃhitā: die saṃhitā der Maitrāyaṇīya-Śākhā. Edited by Leopold von Schroeder. 4 vols. Reprint, Wiesbaden: F. Steiner, 1970–1972.

Manusmṛti, with the commentary of Kullūka Bhaṭṭa. Edited by Gopāla Śāstrī Nene. Kashi Sanskrit Series, no. 114. Varanasi: Chaukhambha Sanskrit Series Office, 1970.

Mārkaṇḍeya Purāṇa. 3 vols. Edited and translated into Hindi by Satyavrat Singh and Mahaprabhulal Goswami. Sitapur: Institute for Puranic and Vedic Studies and Research, 1984–1986.

Matsyapurāṇa, sarala Hindī bhāṣānuvāda sahita. Edited by Śrīrāma Śarmā Āchārya. Barelī: Saṃskṛti Saṃsthāna, 1970.

Padma Purāṇam. 5 vols. Calcutta: Gurumaṇḍalagranthamālā, 18, 1957–1959.

Rāmāyaṇa of Vālmīki. 7 vols. Edited by G. H. Bhatt, et al. Baroda: Oriental Institute, 1960–1975.

Ṛgveda Saṃhitā. Sanskrit text with English translation by Satya Prakash Sarasvati, Satyakam Vidyalankar, and Veda Pratishthana. 13 vols. New Delhi: S. Chand & Co., 1977–1987.

Śabdakalpadrumaḥ. Edited by Rājā Rādhākāntadeva, Varadāprasāda Vasu, and Haricaraṇa Vasu. 5 vols. Reprint, Delhi: Nag Publishers, 2003.

Śakuntalā. Edited with notes by Monier Williams. 2nd ed. Oxford: Clarendon Press, 1876.

Śārṅgadharasaṃhitā, Hṛdayapriyā enna vyākhyānasahitaṃ. Edited by Ānekkāḷīlil Es. Gopālapiḷḷa. 5th ed. Koṭuṅṅallūr: Devi Book Stall, 1998.

Śatapatha Brāhmaṇa in the Mādhyandina-Śākhā, with Extracts from the Commentaries of Sāyaṇa, Harisvāmin, and Dvivedagaṅgā. Edited by Albrecht Weber. Chowkhamba Sanskrit Series, no. 96. Reprint, Benares: Chowkhamba Sanskrit Series Office, 1964.

Śivamahāpurāṇam (samāhātmyam). Edited by Pāṇḍeya Rāmateja. Kāśī: Paṇḍita-Pustakālaya, 1963.

Suśrutasaṃhitā of Suśruta, with the *Nibandhasaṅgraha* of Śrī Ḍalhaṇāchārya and the *Nyāyacandrikā Pañjikā* of Gayadāsāchārya on the Nidānasthāna. Edited by Jādavji Trikamji Āchārya and Nārāyaṇ Rām Āchārya. Jaikrishnadas Ayurveda Series, no. 34. 7th ed. Varanasi: Chaukhambha Orientalia, 2002.

Vāyupurāṇam. Edited by Nārāyaṇa Āpte. Ānandāśrama Sanskrit Series, no. 49. Poona: Anandāśrama-mudraṇālaya, 1905.

Vidyāpariṇayam, Śrīmadānandarāyamakhipraṇītam. Edited by Goparāju Rāmā. Gaṅ-gānāthajhākendrīyasaṃskṛtavidyāpīṭha-granthamālā, no. 30. Allahabad: Gaṅgānāthajhākendrīyasaṃskṛtavidyāpīṭham, 1991.

Vīrasiṃhavalokaḥ, Hindibhāṣānuvāda-vyākhyādirivibhūṣitaḥ, vyākhyākāraḥ Paṇḍita Śrī Rādhākṛṣṇa Pārāśaraḥ. Kṛṣṇadāsa Āyurveda Sīrīja, no. 59. Vārāṇasī: Kṛṣṇadāsa Akādamī, 1999.

Viṣṇupurāṇam. Critical edition and pāda index prepared by M. M. Pathak and Peter Schreiner. Vadodara: Oriental Institute, 1997–1999.

Viṣṇusmṛtiḥ: Śrīnandapaṇḍitaviracitasaṃkṣipta "Vaijantī" vyākhayopetā. Edited by Julius Jolly. Chowkhamba Sanskrit Series, no. 95. Reprint, Vārāṇasī: Caukhambā Saṃskṛta Sīrīja Āphisa, 1962.

Yājñavalkya Smṛti. 2nd ed. Edited by T. Ganapati Sastri. New Delhi: Munshiram Manoharlal, 1982.

Secondary Sources

Agravāla, Saroja. *Prabodhacandrodaya aur uskī Hindī paramparā*. Āgarā Viśvavidyālaya kī Ph.D. Prayāj: Hindī Sāhitya Sammelan, 1962.

Apte, V. S. *Practical Sanskrit-English Dictionary*. 4th ed. Delhi: Motilal Banarsidass, 2004.

Bailey, Greg. *Materials for the Study of Ancient Indian Ideologies:* pravṛtti *and* nivṛtti. Torino: Indologica Taurinensia, 1985.

———. "The *pravṛtti/nivṛtti* project at La Trobe University with Notes on the Meaning of *vṛt* in the *Bhagavadgītā*." *Indologica Taurinensia*, 29 (2003): 9–28.

Bakhśī, Gāyatrī Devī. *Saṃskṛt ke pratīk nāṭak ke rūp meṃ śrī Vedāntadeśika kṛt Saṃkalpasūryodaya ek adhyayan*. Jaipur: Saṃghī Prakāśan, 1993.

Barrett, Ronald L. *Aghor Medicine: Pollution, Death, and Healing in Northern India*. Berkeley: University of California Press, 2008.

Barthes, Roland. *Mythologies*. Translated by Annette Lavers. New York: Hill and Wang, 1972.

Basham, A. L. "The Practice of Medicine in Ancient and Medieval India." In *Asian Medical Systems: A Comparative Study*, edited by Charles Leslie, 18–43. Berkeley: University of California Press, 1976.

Bloomfield, Maurice. *The Atharva-Veda and the Gopatha-Brāhmaṇa (Grundriss der Indo-Arischen Philologie und Altertumskunde)*. Strassburg: Verlag von Karl J. Trübner, 1899.

Bronner, Yigal. *Extreme Poetry: The South Asian Movement of Simultaneous Narration*. New York: Columbia University Press, 2010.

Cappeller, Carl. "Ein Medizinisches Sanskritdrama." In *Festschrift für Ernst Windisch*, 107–115. Leipzig: Harrassowitz, 1914.

Cerulli, Anthony. "Āyurveda." In *Brill's Encyclopedia of Hinduism, Vol. II: Texts, Rituals, Arts, and Concepts*, edited by Knut A. Jacobsen, 267–280. Leiden: Brill Publications, 2010.

———. "Calculating Fecundity in the *Kāśyapa Saṃhitā*." In *Health and Religious Rituals in South Asia: Disease, Possession, and Healing*, edited by Fabrizio Ferrari, 114–126. London: Routledge, 2011.

———. "The Joy of Life: Medicine, Politics, and Religion." In *Medical Texts and Manuscripts in Indian Cultural History*, edited by Anthony Cerulli, Karin Preisendanz, and Dominik Wujastyk. New Delhi: Manohar Publishers, forthcoming.

———. "Religio-Medical Perspectives on the Body, Self, and Embodiment in Āyurveda." In *Refiguring the Body: Embodiment in South Asian Religions*, edited by Barbara Holdrege and Karen Pechilis. Albany: State University of New York Press, forthcoming.

Cerulli, Anthony, and Brahmadathan U. M. T. "Know Thy Body, Know Thyself: Decoding Knowledge of the Ātman in Sanskrit Medical Literature." *Journal of Indian Medicine*, vol. 2, no. 3 (2009): 101–107.

Charon, Rita. *Narrative Medicine: Honoring the Stories of Illness*. New York: Oxford University Press, 2006.

Charon, Rita, and Martha Montello, eds., *Stores Matter: The Role of Narrative in Medical Ethics*. New York: Routledge, 2002.

Chattopadhyaya, Debiprasad. "Tradition of Rationalist Medicine in Ancient India: Case for a Critical Analysis of the *Caraka-saṃhitā*." In *Sanskrit and World Culture: Proceedings of the Fourth World Sanskrit Conference of the International Association of Sanskrit Studies*, edited by Wolfgang Morgenworth, 85–115. Berlin: Akademie-Verlag, 1986.

Comba, Antonella. "Carakasaṃhitā, Śārīrasthāna I and Vaiśeṣika Philosophy." In *Studies on Indian Medical History* (1987), edited by G. Jan Meulenbeld and Dominik Wujastyk, 39–55. Reprint, Delhi: Motilal Banarsidass, 2001.

Cordier, Palmyr. *Étude sur la Médecine Hindoue: (Temps Védiques et Héroiques)*. Thèse pour le Doctorat en Médecine, Faculté de Médecine et de Pharmacie de Bordeaux. Paris: A. Bellier et Ce., 1894.

Das, Rahul Peter. "Notions of 'Contagion' in Classical Indian Medical Texts." In *Contagion: Perspectives from Pre-Modern Societies*, edited by Lawrence I. Conrad and Dominik Wujastyk, 55–78. Aldershot: Ashgate Publishing, 2000.

———. *The Origin of the Life of a Human Being: Conception and the Female According to Ancient Indian Medical and Sexological Literature*. Delhi: Motilal Banarsidass, 2003.

Dasgupta, Surendranath. *A History of Indian Philosophy*, vol. II. 5th ed. London: Cambridge University Press, 1968.

Dash, Bhagwan, and Lalitesh Kasyap. *Five Specialised Therapies of Ayurveda (Pañca-karma)*. New Delhi: Concept Publishing Company, 1992.

Dimmit, Cornelia, and J. A. B. van Buitenen. *Classical Hindu Mythology. A Reader in the Sanskrit Purāṇas*. Philadelphia: Temple University Press, 1978.

Doniger, Wendy. "Minimyths and Maximyths and Political Points of View." In *Myth and Method*, edited by Laurie L. Patton and Wendy Doniger, 109–127. Charlottesville: University Press of Virginia, 1996.

Doniger, Wendy, and Sudhir Kakar, trans. *Kamasutra*. Oxford: Oxford University Press, 2002.

Dormandy, Thomas. *The White Death: A History of Tuberculosis*. New York: New York University Press, 2000.

Dubos, René J., and Jean Dubos. *The White Plague: Tuberculosis, Man, and Society*, 1952. Reprint, New Brunswick: Rutgers University Press, 1987.

Engler, Steven. "'Science' vs. 'Religion' in Classical Ayurveda." *Numen*, vol. 50 (2003): 416–463.

Filliozat, Jean. *Etude de démonologie indienne. Le Kumāratantra de Rāvaṇa et les textes parallèles indiens, tibétains, chinois, cambodgien et arabe.* Paris: Imprimerie Nationale, 1937.

———. *The Classical Doctrine of Indian Medicine: Its Origins and Greek Parallels.* Translated by Dev Raj Chanana. Delhi: Munshiram Manoharlal, 1964.

Foucault, Michel. *The Birth of the Clinic: An Archaeology of Medical Perception.* Translated by A. M. Sheridan Smith. New York: Vintage Books, 1973.

Geertz, Clifford. *The Interpretation of Cultures.* New York: Basic Books, 1973.

Gonda, Jan. *Change and Continuity in Indian Religion*, 1965. Reprint, New Delhi: Munshiram Manoharlal, 1997.

Grotenhuis, Elizabeth Ten. *Along the Silk Road.* Washington, DC: Arthur M. Sackler Gallery, Smithsonian Institute, 2002.

Hara, Minoru. "A Note on the Buddha's Birth Story." In *Indianisme et Bouddhisme: Mélanges offerts à Mgr Étienne Lamotte*, 143–157. Louvain: Université Catholique de Louvain, 1980.

Heesterman, J. C. *The Ancient Indian Royal Consecration: The Rājāsūya Described according to the Yajus Texts.* Disputationes Rheno-trajectinae 2. 's-Gravenhage: Mouton, 1957.

Hoernle, A. F. Rudolf. *Studies in the Medicine of Ancient India: Part I, Osteology or the Bones of the Human Body.* Oxford: Clarendon Press, 1907.

Jamison, Stephanie. *Sacrificed Wife/Sacrificer's Wife: Women, Ritual, and Hospitality in Ancient India.* Oxford: Oxford University Press, 1996.

Jolly, Julius. *Indian Medicine.* Translated by C. G. Kashikar. 3rd ed. New Delhi: Munshiram Manoharlal, 1994.

Kakar, Sudhir. *The Inner World: A Psycho-analytic Study of Childhood and Society in India.* 2nd ed. Delhi: Oxford University Press, 1981.

Kapani, Lakshmi. "Note on the Garbha-Upaniṣad." In *Fragments for a History of the Human Body*, edited by Michel Feher, Ramona Naddaff, and Nadia Tazi, 181–196. Zone 5, Part III. New York: Zone Books, 1989.

Kapani, Lakshmi, trans. "Upaniṣad of the Embryo." In *Fragments for a History of the Human Body*, edited by Michel Feher, Ramona Naddaff, and Nadia Tazi, 177–179. Zone 5, Part III. New York: Zone Books, 1989.

Kapstein, Matthew T., trans. *The Rise of Wisdom Moon by Krishna-mishra.* New York: New York University Press and JJC Foundation, 2009.

Kaul, Advaitavadini, and Utpal Kaul. "Wisdom of Kashmir—The Assimilator of Knowledge Channels." In *Kashmiri Pandits: Looking to the Future*, edited by M. K. Kaw, 85–92. New Delhi: Kashmir Education, Culture and Science Society, 2001.

Kuppuswami Sastri, T. S. "Ramabhadra-Dikshita and the Southern Poets of His Time." *Indian Antiquary*, vol. 33. (May 1904): 126–142, 176–196.

Lacey, Louise. *Lunaception: A Feminine Odyssey into Fertility and Contraception.* New York: Coward, McCann, and Geoghegen, 1975.

Lanman, Charles Rockwell. *A Sanskrit Reader, with Vocabulary and Notes*, parts I and II. London: Trübner & Co., Ludgate Hill, 1884.

Larson, Gerald. "Karma as a 'Sociology of Knowledge' or 'Social Psychology' of Process / Praxis." In *Karma and Rebirth in Classical Indian Traditions* (1980), edited by Wendy Doniger O'Flaherty, 303–316. Reprint, Delhi: Motilal Banarsidass, 1983.

———. "Āyurveda and the Hindu Philosophical Systems." *Philosophy East and West*, vol. 37, no. 3 (July 1987): 245–259.

———. *Classical Sāṃkhya: An Interpretation of Its History and Meaning*. 5th ed. Delhi: Motilal Banarsidass, 2005.

Lévi-Strauss, Claude. *The Jealous Potter*. Chicago: University of Chicago Press, 1988.

Lochan, Kanjiv. *Medicines of Early India*. Varanasi: Chaukhambha Sanskrit Bhawan, 2003.

Lupton, Deborah. *Medicine as Culture: Illness, Disease and the Body in Western Societies*. 2nd ed. London: Sage Publications, 2004.

Maas, Philipp. "On What Became of the *Carakasaṃhitā* after Dṛḍhabala's Revision." *Journal of Indian Medicine*, vol. 3 (2010): 1–22.

MacIntyre, Alasdair. *After Virtue: A Study in Moral Virtue*. South Bend: University of Notre Dame Press, 1981.

Malamoud, Charles. *Cooking the World: Ritual & Thought in Ancient India*. Translated by David White. Delhi: Oxford University Press, 1996.

Malandra, Geri. *Unfolding a Maṇḍala: The Buddhist Cave Temples at Ellora*. Albany: State University of New York Press, 1993.

Marriott, McKim. "Hindu Transactions: Diversity without Dualism." In *Transaction and Meaning: Directions in the Anthropology of Exchange and Symbolic Behavior*, edited by B. Kapferer, 109–142. Philadelphia: Institute for the Study of Human Issues, 1976.

Matilal, Bimal Krishna. "Scepticism and Mysticism." *Journal of the American Oriental Society*, vol. 105, no. 3 (1985): 479–484.

Mattingly, Cheryl. "In Search of the Good: Narrative Reasoning in Clinical Practice." *Medical Anthropology Quarterly*, 12/3 (1998): 273–297.

Mauss, Marcel. "Techniques of the Body." Translated by Ben Brewster. *Economy and Society*, vol, 2, no. 1 (February, 1973): 70–87.

Mazars, Guy. *A Concise Introduction to Indian Medicine (La Médecine indienne)*. Translated by T. K. Gopalan. Delhi: Motilal Banarsidass, 2006.

Meulenbeld, Gerrit Jan. *A History of Indian Medical Literature*. 5 vols. Groningen: E. Forsten, 1999–2002.

———. "The Woes of *Ojas* in the Modern World." In *Modern and Global Ayurveda: Pluralism and Paradigms*, edited by Dagmar Wujastyk and Frederick M. Smith, 157–175. Albany: State University of New York Press, 2008.

Meulenbeld, G. Jan, and Dominik Wujastyk, ed. *Studies on Indian Medical History*, 1987. Reprint, Delhi: Motilal Banarsidass, 2001.

Monier-Williams, Monier. *Hinduism*. London: Society for Promoting Christian Knowledge, 1880.

Monier-Williams, Monier, ed. *Sanskrit-English Dictionary: Etymologically and Philologically Arranged With Special Reference to Cognate Indo-European Languages*, 1899. Reprint, Delhi: Motilal Banarsidass, 1997.

Mukhopadhyaya, Girindranath. *History of Indian Medicine*. 3 vols, 1923. Reprint, New Delhi: Munshiram Manoharlal, 1994.

O'Flaherty, Wendy Doniger. *Śiva: The Erotic Ascetic*. Oxford: Oxford University Press, 1973.

———. *Hindu Myths: A Sourcebook Translated from the Sanskrit*. London: Penguin Books, 1975.

———. *The Origins of Evil in Hindu Mythology*. Berkeley: University of California Press, 1976.

———. *Women, Androgynes, and Other Mythical Beasts*. Chicago: University of Chicago Press, 1980.

———. "Karma and Rebirth in the Vedas and Purāṇas." In *Karma and Rebirth in Classical Indian Traditions* (1980), edited by Wendy Doniger O'Flaherty, 3–37. Reprint, Delhi: Motilal Banarsidass, 1983.

———. *Tales of Sex and Violence: Folklore, Sacrifice, and Danger in the Jaiminīya Brāhmaṇa*. Chicago: University of Chicago Press, 1985.

O'Flaherty, Wendy Doniger, ed. *Karma and Rebirth in Classical Indian Traditions*, 1980. Reprint, Delhi: Motilal Banarsidass, 1983.

Olivelle, Patrick. *The Āśrama System: The History and Hermeneutics of a Religious Institution*, 1993. Reprint, New Delhi: Munshiram Manoharlal, 2004.

Olivelle, Patrick, trans. *Upaniṣads*. New York: Oxford University Press, 1996.

Perry, Edward Delavan. *A Sanskrit Primer Based on the Leitfaden für den Elementar-Cursus des Sanskrit of Professor Georg Bühler of Vienna*. Boston: Ginn and Company, 1885.

Pintchman, Tracy. *The Rise of the Goddess in the Hindu Tradition*. Albany: State University of New York Press, 1994.

Pollock, Sheldon. "Rāmāyaṇa and Political Imagination in India." *Journal of Asian Studies*, vol. 52, no. 2 (May 1993): 261--297.

———. *The Language of the Gods in the World of Men: Sanskrit, Culture, and Power in Premodern India*, 2006. Reprint, Delhi: Permanent Black, 2007.

Pollock, Sheldon, et al. "Sanskrit Knowledge Systems on the Eve of Colonialism Project." 2001–2004. http://www.columbia.edu/itc/mealac/pollock/sks/index.html.

Preisendanz, Karin. "Mahābhūtas." In *Brill's Encyclopedia of Hinduism, Vol. II: Texts, Rituals, Arts, and Concepts*, edited by Knut A. Jacobsen, 806–818. Leiden: Brill Publications, 2010.

Raghavan, V., ed. *Śāhendravilāsa (A Poem on the Life of King Śāhaji of Tanjore, 1684–1710) of Śrīdhara Veṅkaṭeśa (Ayyāvāl)*. Tañjapurī Sarasvatīmahālaya-granthamālā, no. 54. Tanjore: T.M.S.S.M. Library, 1952.

Ramanujan, A. K. "Is There an Indian Way of Thinking?" In *India Through Hindu Categories*, edited by McKim Marriott, 41–58. New Delhi: Sage Publications, 1990.

Roşu, Arion. "Etudes âyurvédiques III: Les carrés magiques dans la médecine indienne." In *Studies on Indian Medical History* (1987), edited by G. Jan

Meulenbeld and Dominik Wujastyk, 95–104. Reprint, Delhi: Motilal Banarsidass, 2001.

Ryan, Frank. *The Forgotten Plague: How the Battle against Tuberculosis was Won—and Lost*. Boston: Little, Brown and Company, 1992.

Scharfe, Hartmut. "The Doctrine of the Three Humors in Traditional Indian Medicine and the Alleged Antiquity of Tamil Siddha Medicine." *Journal of the American Oriental Society*, vol. 119, no. 4 (October–December 1999): 609–629.

Schetelich, Maria. "Niti in Anandarayamakhis Drama 'Jivanandana.'" *Altorientalische Forschungen*, 11.2 (1984): 299–330.

Selby, Martha Ann. "Narratives of Conception, Gestation, and Labour in Sanskrit Ayurvedic Texts." *Asian Medicine: Tradition and Modernity*, vol. 1, no. 2 (2005): 254–275.

Sharma, P. V. "Other Compendia of *Bhela, Kāśyapa*, and *Hārīta*." In *History of Medicine in India: From Antiquity to 1000 A.D.*, edited by P. V. Sharma, 223–228. New Delhi: Indian National Science Academy, 1992.

———. *Rogī-parīkṣa-vidhi*, 1957. V. Āyurevda-granthamālā, no. 15. Reprint, Vārāṇasī: Caukhambhā Bhāratī Akādamī, 2003.

———. *Āyurved kā Vaijñānik Itihās*. 7th ed. Jaikrishnadas Ayurveda Series, no. 1. Benares: Chowkhamba Orientalia, 2003.

Sharma, P. V., ed. *History of Medicine in India: From Antiquity to 1000 A.D.* New Delhi: Indian National Science Academy, 1992.

Shekhar, I. *Sanskrit Drama: Its Origin and Decline*. Leiden: E.J. Brill, 1960.

Sircar, D. C. *The Śākta Pīṭhas*. 2nd ed. Delhi: Motilal Banarsidass, 1973.

Smith, Brian K. *Classifying the Universe: The Ancient Indian Varṇa System and the Origins of Caste*. Oxford: Oxford University Press, 1994.

Srikanta Murthy, K. R. "Suśruta." In *History of Medicine in India: From Antiquity to 1000 A.D.*, edited by P. V. Sharma, 197–204. New Delhi: Indian National Science Academy, 1992.

Staal, J. F., ed. *A Reader on the Sanskrit Grammarians*. Cambridge, MA: The MIT Press, 1972.

Subramanian, K.R. *The Maratha Rajas of Tanjore*. Madras: K. R. Subramanian, 1928.

Taussig, Michael. "Reification and the Consciousness of the Patient." *Social Science & Medicine*. Part B, Medical Anthropology. Vol. 14B, no. 1 (February 1980): 3–13.

Tewari, Premvati V. *Introduction to Kāśyapa-Saṃhitā*. Varanasi: Chaukhambha Visvabharati, 1997.

———. *Āyurvedīya Prasūtitantra Evaṃ Strītoga*. 2 vols. 3rd ed. Varanasi: Chaukhambha Orientalia, 2003.

Thapar, Romila. *Time as a Metaphor of History: The Krishna Bharadwaj Memorial Lecture*. New Delhi: Oxford University Press, 1996.

———. *Early India: From the Origins to AD 1300*. London: Penguin Press, 2002.

Valiathan, M. S. *The Legacy of Caraka*. Chennai: Orient Longman, 2003.

Vallauri, Mario, trans. *Jīvānandana (La Felicità Dell' Anima) di Ānandarāyamakhin*. Lanciano: G. Carabba, 1929.

Varier, N. V. Krishnankutty. *History of Ayurveda*. Kottakkal Ayurveda Series, 56. Kottakkal: Arya Vaidya Sala Publications, 2005.

Veyne, Paul. *Did the Greeks Believe in Their Myths: An Essay on the Constitutive Imagination*. Translated by Paula Wissing. Chicago: University of Chicago Press, 1988.

Weckerling, Adolf, trans. *Das Glück des Lebens: Medizinisches Drama von Ânandarâyamakhî*. Greifswald: Universitätsverlag Ratsbuchandlung L. Bamberg, 1937.

Weiss, Mitchell. "Caraka Saṃhitā on the Doctrine of Karma." In *Karma and Rebirth in Classical Indian Traditions* (1980), edited by Wendy Doniger O'Flaherty, 90–115. Reprint, Delhi: Motilal Banarsidass, 1983.

White, David Gordon. *The Alchemical Body: Siddha Traditions in Medieval India*. Chicago: University of Chicago Press, 1996.

———. *Kiss of the Yoginī: "Tantric Sex" in Its South Asian Contexts*. Chicago: University of Chicago Press, 2003.

Whitney, William Dwight. *A Sanskrit Grammar, including both the Classical Language and the Older Dialects, of Veda and Brahmana*. 17th ed. Cambridge, MA: Harvard University Press, 1993.

Wilkins, W. J. *Hindu Mythology, Vedic and Purāṇic*, 1882. Reprint, Varanasi: Indological Book House, 1972.

Wood, Frances. *The Silk Road: Two Thousand Years in the Heart of Asia*. Berkeley: University of California Press, 2002.

Woodburne, A. Stewart. "The Evil Eye in South Indian Folklore." In *The Evil Eye: A Casebook*, edited by Alan Dundes, 55–65. Madison: University of Wisconsin Press, 1981.

Wujastyk, Dagmar. *Well-Mannered Medicine: Medical Ethics and Etiquette in Classical Ayurveda*. New York: Oxford University Press, 2012.

Wujastyk, Dominik. "Miscarriages of Justice: Demonic Vengeance in Classical Indian Medicine." In *Religion, Health, and Suffering*, edited by J. Hinnels and R. Porter, 256–275. London: Kegan Paul International, 1999.

———. "Interpréter l' Image du Corps Humain dans l' Inde Pré-Moderne." In *Images du corps dans le monde hindou*, edited by Véronique Bouillier and Gilles Tarabout, 71–99. Paris: CNRS-Éditions, 2002.

———. *The Roots of Ayurveda: Selections from Sanskrit Medical Writings*. 3rd ed. London: Penguin Books, 2003.

———. "The Science of Medicine." In *The Blackwell Companion to Hinduism*, edited by Gavin Flood, 393–409. Malden, MA: Blackwell Publishing, 2003.

———. "Medicine and Dharma." *Journal of Indian Philosophy*, vol. 32 (2004): 831–842.

———. Review of *A History of Indian Medical Literature*, by G. Jan Meulenbeld, *Bulletin of the School of Oriental and African Studies*, University of London, vol. 67, no. 3 (2004): 404–407.

———. "Regulation of Āyurveda in Great Britain in the Twenty-First Century." *Asian Medicine: Tradition and Modernity*, vol. 1, no. 1 (2005): 162–184.

———. "The Questions of King Tukkoji: Medicine at an Eighteenth Century South Indian Court." *Indian Journal of History of Science,* 41.4 (2006): 357–369.

Yamashita, Tsutomu. "Śārīrasthāna of the Āyurveda—A Comparative Study." *Studies in the History of Indian Thought,* vol. 7 (1995): 105–113.

———. "Towards a Critical Edition of the *Bhelasaṃhitā.*" *Journal of the European Ayurvedic Society,* vol. 5 (1997): 19–24.

Zimmer, Heinrich. *Hindu Medicine,* 1948. Reprint, New York: Arno Press, 1979.

Zimmermann, Francis. "Remarks on the Conception of the Body in Ayurvedic Medicine." *South Asian Digest of Regional Writing,* vol. 8 (1979): 10–26.

———. "Ṛtu-Sātmya: The Seasonal Cycle and the Principle of Appropriateness." Translated by M. Marriott and J. Leavitt. *Social Science & Medicine.* Part B, Medical Anthropology. Vol. 14B, no. 2 (May 1980): 99–106.

———. "Terminological Problems in the Process of Editing and Translating Sanskrit Medical Texts." In *Approaches to Traditional Chinese Medical Literature,* edited by Paul Unschuld, 141–151. Dordrecht: Kluwer Academic, 1989.

———. *The Jungle and the Aroma of Meats: An Ecological Theme in Hindu Medicine,* 1987 (orig. French pub., 1982). Reprint, Delhi: Motilal Banarsidass, 1999.

———. "'May Godly Clouds Rain For You!': Metaphors of Well-Being in Sanskrit." *Studia Asiatica,* V (2004): 1–12.

Zysk, Kenneth G. "Fever in Vedic India." *Journal of the American Oriental Society,* vol. 103, no. 3 (July–September 1983): 617–621.

———. "The Evolution of Anatomical Knowledge in Ancient India, with Special Reference to Cross-Cultural Influences." *Journal of the American Oriental Society,* vol. 106, no. 4 (October–December 1986): 687–705.

———. *Asceticism and Healing in Ancient India: Medicine in the Buddhist Monastery.* Oxford: Oxford University Press, 1991.

———. *Medicine in the Veda: Religious Healing in the Veda,* 1985. Reprint, Delhi: Motilal Banarsidass, 1996.

———. "Does Ancient Indian Medicine Have a Theory of Contagion?" In *Contagion: Perspectives from Pre-Modern Societies,* edited by Lawrence I. Conrad and Dominik Wujastyk, 79–95. Aldershot: Ashgate Publishing, 2000.

———. "Potency Therapy in Classical Indian Medicine." *Asian Medicine: Tradition and Modernity,* vol. 1, no. 1 (2005): 101–118.

Index